THE WELLBEING REVOLUTION

Mastering **Extraordinary** Human Living

James McWhinney

Copyright © 2011 by James McWhinney

All Rights Reserved. No part of this publication may be reproduced in any form or by any means, including scanning, photocopying, or otherwise without prior written permission of the copyright holder.

ISBN 978-0-9872150-0-0

Edited by Judith Ashby
Book design by Carla Green

Contents

THE WELLBEING REVOLUTION BEGINS NOW 1

SPIRITUALITY 15

Life's Greatest Lesson #1
EVERYTHING IS CONNECTED 19

Life's Greatest Lesson #2
EVERYTHING HAPPENS FOR A REASON 25

Life's Greatest Lesson #3
EVERYTHING HAS A PURPOSE 39
    Life's Greatest Gift – Universal Energy 47
    Discovering What Really Creates Wellbeing 62
    Effects of Low Energy 69

FULFILLING YOUR POTENTIAL 84

FINDING YOUR PURPOSE 89
    Discovering Your Greatest Passions 94
    Discovering Your Greatest Strengths 98
    Discovering Your Deepest Values 102
    Discovering Your Deepest Desires 105
    Discovering Your Greatest Inspirations and Motivations 106
    Discovering Your Spiritual Essence 107

FURTHER CONNECTING TO ENERGY ... 110
- Live in the Present Moment ... 111
- Integrity ... 122
- Meditation ... 128
- Gratitude ... 144
- Love What You Do ... 150
- Love Your Unique Self ... 154
- Connect to Service ... 163
- Connecting With Others Through Giving ... 164
- Connect to Nature ... 170
- Eat Healthily ... 170
- Exercise ... 172
- Breathe Deeply ... 173

HOW TO OVERCOME OBSTACLES ALONG YOUR JOURNEY ... 175

HAPPY JOURNEY! ... 185

ABOUT JAMES McWHINNEY ... 187

The Wellbeing Revolution Begins Now

"Your time is limited, so don't waste it living someone else's life. Don't be trapped by dogma — which is living with the results of other people's thinking. Don't let the noise of others' opinions drown out your own inner voice. And most important, have the courage to follow your heart and intuition. They somehow already know what you truly want to become. Everything else is secondary."
— Steve Jobs, Stanford Commencement Speech 2005.

The wellbeing revolution begins now. Your wellbeing is dependent on your willingness to courageously flaunt your unique inner drive. Yes, you have a unique inner drive, and the quality of your life is determined by your compliance and manner in which you fully give it to the world. This book has been specifically written to help you create an extraordinary life, a life that frees you to do whatever you want, whenever you want — a life truly worth living.

Have you ever noticed that near-death experiences are the greatest catalyst for change in people's lives? You may know certain people who faced the prospect of death, only to come through the experience with a profoundly new attitude to the way they want to live. These people create a great shift, changing their priorities and perspective on the world and those around them. It's as though people only really start to live when they face death and with this new attitude they embrace life fully without holding back. They treat their lives and the lives of those around them with much more vigour, excitement and love. Instead of working harder at their jobs, they work harder on themselves. Instead of wasting their time in meaningless and unimportant pursuits, they live every moment as though it is a gift.

Since too few people figure out what they want from life before it's too late, I'm here to tell you that you don't need to face death before you truly start living the great life that you were born to live. I'm going to help you create an incredible life without having to hear that you have one month to live before an illness takes you over. I will enable you to discover a new perspective on your life, whilst at the same time assisting you to discover your true potential.

This book could mark the most significant turning-point of your life through its discussion of one the most important universal truths known to man. It is aimed at opening your mind to discovering your unique inner drive so that you may live an incredible life, reaching your infinite potential full of possibilities and meaning. I'm going to explain to you that each and every single person on this earth is born with a unique purpose and call of their soul during their lifetime, and that by connecting to the energy of the world and fulfilling that purpose you are capable of living the life that you are truly meant to live. Within this book lies the greatest strategy to remove yourself from a life of constant stress and struggles and restore you to living a pleasurable, purposeful and meaningful life.

This book has not been written for the average person, or the person who is willing to accept a life of mediocrity; it has been written for those who seek to live an incredible life full of consistent happiness, love, fulfillment and meaning – for those who seek the courage to follow their destiny. From this very moment forward you must commit to living your life at its absolute highest level.

As a global society, we've totally lost ourselves in trying to enhance our situation by creating **bigger, better** and **more**: more wealth, more possessions, more power, more status. We've lost ourselves in creating extrinsic security to the point where people neglect the entire point of their existence. Working more hours in order to have more 'things' has become of paramount importance to the majority of people in this world. Yet, have you noticed the exorbitant amount of people who loath their jobs? I don't think the words 'Thank God it's Monday' have ever been said seriously. It seems that 99% of the world want to *escape* from their current life. Does this sound like you? Do you feel your current position in life makes full use of your abilities? Do you feel fully expressed every single day?

We're hurting ourselves, we're hurting one another and we're hurting the world.

Our world's values are dissipating and we need to wake up from our current way of living. People are searching for happiness and meaning through money, status and power and are consequently becoming *much less* happy. Depression is quickly becoming one of the world's most common illnesses and people have lost sight of what is truly important.

Have you taken a moment to question why the world has been hit with many deadly natural disasters throughout the last decade? You may believe the reason to be cyclical or even the consequence of global warming. I strongly believe there is greater meaning behind such 'disasters'. The world's intelligent system is trying to wake us up from the collective dysfunction of society. Take a moment to think about the negative impact we have on the world. We're killing animals to the point of extinction for *profit*. We're cutting down the world's natural habitats and rainforests for *profit*. We're destroying the earth by drilling deeper and deeper for...you guessed it, *profit*. Collectively, people value money more that they value the amazing world that was *created* for each and every one of us. Continually proven by many scientists and psychologists, money will not bring you lasting happiness, yet it's as though most people believe that making money is the only means to creating happiness in their lives. Our desire for more money masks a need for something much deeper – *universal energy* – which I will discuss later. We have enough resources to be 'comfortable' beyond our need, yet driven by greed and fear we are continually exploiting our natural resources to the point that the Higher Power of this incredible world is forcing us to wake up and change our ways.

In a drive to acquire more energy, people have become more concerned about making themselves feel significant than helping others. The alarmingly high rates of Botox, facial surgery, breast implants and liposuction prove that we are becoming more concerned with ourselves and our appearance than we are in classic values such as love, giving to and caring about our community – values that we all know aid happiness and fulfillment. As well as indifference, *greed* and *selfishness* caused by fear and insecurity are slowly destroying our lives. You need only take a look at the global economy to notice this. Our once highly held values have increasingly become neglected and consequently the amazing world that we live in is suffering.

Rather than being fuelled by the most fulfilling sensation of giving our greatest selves to others, we're fuelled by ego and selfishness. Rather than focusing on the beauty of the present moment, we incessantly think about the failures of our past and the anxieties of our future, causing stress, fear, worry, anger, anxiety and resentment. Rather than accepting the greatness that surrounds us and finding pleasure in the little things, we continually resist everything and search for reasons to complain.

The world has reached the point where collectively people will only either awaken through suffering or a change in consciousness. Simply, we need to stop interfering and going against what Universal Intelligence – the creator of this world – has made for us. One hopes that something really bad doesn't have to happen for the people of the world to change their consciousness. To awaken, however, is to realise what is most important, to realise the significance of purpose and to replace obstructive values and attitudes with positive values and attitudes that allow you to live your life to its fullest potential.

People are already suffering, feeling emotions that are not favourable to being well and living lives that are void of meaning. Do you suffer from incessant worry, stress, fear, unhappiness and/or depression? If so, your certainly not alone. At the rate we are going the world will continue to suffer until people feel forced to make a change. Just as a smoker is forced to quit smoking when he is told that he has developed lung cancer, the world will need to feel intense suffering before it changes its ways.

As we awaken and realise what is truly important, we'll realise that working over forty hours per week in a job we don't really like in order to accumulate more money, possessions, power and status *doesn't make sense* and is simply the workings of the fear-based egoic mind. We'll discover that the current dysfunction of the world is caused by egotism and we'll learn to release emphasis on that which is unimportant and will instead discover the value of fulfilling our purpose, helping others, finding inner peace, enjoying the present moment and loving one another unconditionally. When eventually we have created so much suffering that we are forced to change our ways, we will revert to what is truly important and find what truly brings us happiness. But this doesn't need to happen.

As we re-establish our values and once again discover what is truly important, the shell of the ego will crack and we will become able to find deeper meaning in ourselves and our world. We will surrender to what is and find meaningful peace and happiness within.

Years ago, I came across this quote from J. Kyle Howard, a prominent self growth authority[1]. The quote still holds true to this day.

"Isn't it amazing that the one thing that should be of the utmost importance to us, our lives, is often the one thing that we understand least. We study to become doctors, lawyers, etc. yet we spend little to no time trying to understand ourselves. Sure we listen to the experts who tell us who we are and what we should be. We are born in to the expectations of other people. From day one, someone who has little to no knowledge of themselves, decides who and what we should be."

Do you know who you truly are and what the motivating factors are behind everything that you do in your life? If you want to live an incredible life it is imperative that you know who you truly are and to do so you must explore who you truly are. This is the most important information that you will ever acquire because your unique internal drive determines your ability to fulfill your potential, which in turn determines the quality of your life; this is more important than anything else. After all, the extent to which you know yourself establishes the quality of the relationships which you can have with others.

Who are you? Are you a nurse, a banker, a student, a tradesperson, a salesperson or a corporate worker? No, that is not who you are. That is simply the role that you define yourself by. Who you truly are runs much deeper than that. The role you define yourself by only obscures your unique, true self. If you don't know who you are and what drives you, it's likely you'll live the life that **other** people want you to live; a shallow existence of unfulfilled potential. I emphasise potential because quite simply the level to which you fulfill your potential determines the quality of your life. Your time on earth will not be fulfilling if you live your life based on what will make others happy because you won't be fulfilling your potential. It is impossible to live life on your own terms if you don't take the time to discover who you truly are. So I ask you, how often do you reflect on the person that you are? How often do you account for your thoughts and actions? If this is not a practice that you are currently familiar with, I guarantee that your life will take a huge positive shift when you begin this process of introspection.

---

1 http://www.define-your-purpose-in-life.com/

Throughout this book you will learn that you have been created uniquely, unlike any other person in this world. Once you begin to discover who you are, what you stand for and the gifts that you have been blessed with, you will be in a position to live a life of meaning, to fulfill your purpose and create greatness in the world. It's so important to 'know thyself,'[2] for if you don't, you will live a meaningless life in a constant search for fulfillment. If you don't *know yourself* you'll spend your life unconsciously chasing things that you think will make you happy such as money, relationships, status and power, and unfortunately will never achieve lasting meaning, happiness or wellbeing in your life.

It's highly likely that who you think you are and what you stand for are not who you truly are, but is in fact who your parents, peers and society want you to be. People who often have little to no knowledge of themselves decide who and what we should be. Don't you think it's crazy that we become certain people and spend our lives chasing things that we are told are important, when the people who told us who we should be and what we should strive for were uninformed to begin with? Each and every single person begins life as a free spirit but slowly gets smothered and told 'who to be' by people who think they know what is right for us, when generally these people don't even know what is right for themselves. It is little wonder that so many people are currently living lives feeling void of meaning when you discover that each and every person's true self has been smothered and confined to what society thinks it should be. You were born to be *you*, not who society wants you to be. Allowing your life to be guided by external influences rather than your hearts true desires is the cause of any problem that you will ever encounter throughout your lifetime. You can do far better than this.

Most of us spend up to ten hours a day doing something that we don't really like. Not only are most people not fulfilling their highest potential, which is *the number one guarantee to live a fulfilling life*, some people even go against their own personal values in order to keep the pay coming in. Many people are very selective when it comes to their life partner, yet they will spend a third of their life doing a job that they don't really like. So many people are obsessed with their work that they de-

---

2 *Know thyself* is an Ancient Greek aphorism – inscribed at the Temple of Apollo at Delphi. Employed by Plato, this wisdom is thought to be a command from the Ancient Greek Gods.

velop stress related illnesses and diseases. Their work has become all consuming, a facade masking their true feelings and desires and which aids the neglect of life's most important question: 'Why am I here?' Yet, people are unwilling to slow down and are in a continual push to have, and be, more, seeking only to enhance themselves in the eyes of others.

The time has come for you to stop compromising your life; to stop waking up begrudgingly to your alarm clock every morning, rustling in bed until it gets to the point where if you don't get up you know you're going to be late; to stop reluctantly getting up and making your way to work because you *have* to, not because you *want* to; to stop spending most of the day checking the clock, counting the hours until you can finally go home, only to eat dinner, watch boring television and then go to bed dreading waking up to do the same thing the following morning – and then again the next day, and the next, and the next, for the rest of your life. If you feel stuck in your situation, know that this is a toxic way to live. This is a life of restricted energy and unfulfilled potential. To spend your life in this way is to miss the point of human existence. This mediocre, meaningless mode of survival is what causes the majority of the world to search for refuge and try to escape their daily lives through excessive consumption of alcohol, drugs, food, television, fashion and sex. The steady increase of attempted escapism through over consumption of such 'remedies' in today's world is causing escalated levels of unhappiness, anxiety, stress, worry and depression.

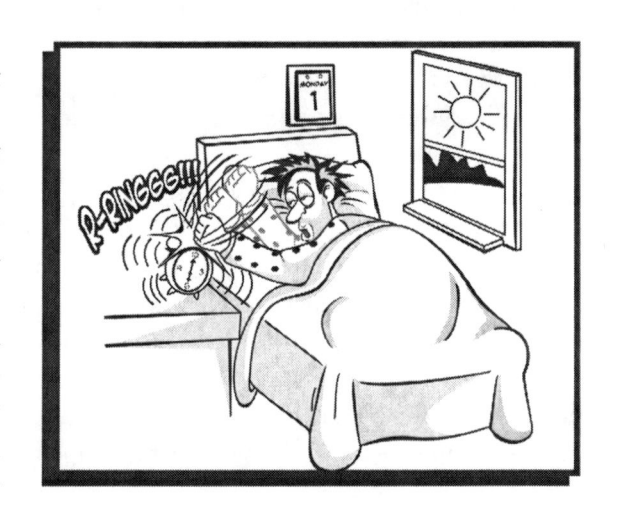

It's safe to assume that you've been living your life a certain way for the past number of years. After all, humans are creatures of habit. I want you to ask yourself right now if you are happy with the way your life is progressing, if you're 100% happy with the life that you are living right now, not 'one day' in the future but now. Is your life full of meaning? Are you fully expressing yourself, or do you feel stuck, trapped and craving an escape?

If you are ready to change your life, there are some important steps that you're going to need to take. These steps provide the *only known methods* to creating an amazing life – but you can't expect to live a happy, loving, meaningful life if all you do is idly wish or dream about it. You must be willing to do the required work to create positive changes in your life.

Step one: Heightening your sense of spirituality

To heighten your spirituality, I will help you to understand that:
1. Everything is connected
2. Everything happens for a reason
3. Everything has a purpose

Quite simply, heightening your sense of spirituality will align yourself with what nature has created you for. You will learn that it doesn't matter how much money, power, status or possessions you acquire, your life will not be fulfilling until you align yourself with this spiritual power. After all, how can you ever give your whole heart to living your life if you can't see the bigger picture? As you align yourself to the same power and energy that created you and the world you live in, you will enjoy consistent happiness regardless of what is happening in your life.

Step two: Discovering that you have a unique inner drive

The quality of your life is determined by your ability to fully give to the world that which you are most driven by. This section will discuss the significance of giving your greatest self to the world and provide you with essential exercises that you need to take to fulfill your greatest potential.

Step three: Finding the answer to life's biggest question – 'Why am I here?'

This step provides activities that will allow you to find your true self, and in doing so, help you to discover why you've been born into this great world. I'm not talking about the 'self' that others demand you to be or the self that acts a certain way to fit in and conform with what society accepts, I'm talking about the true you, the you who is craving to authentically express your special and unique qualities to the world. By tapping into your subconscious you will discover your unique passions, strengths, values and desires, which are all yearning for your expression. You have a unique purpose and once you align yourself with your purpose you will begin to see real magic in your life.

Step four: Activities to enhance your life

This step provides numerous activities that will bring you to peak health and wellbeing and allow you to be at your absolute best both physically and spiritually so that you have the required energy to create the life that you are truly meant to live.

Step five: Overcoming obstacles along your journey

This step is vital in helping you to gain the courage needed to escape your current circumstances and allow you to fully give your deepest inner drive to the world despite any obstacles that may get in your way. I will bust the myths and fears that hold you back from the being able to consistently do what you love and allow you to express your greatest self through greatest service to the world.

Combined, these steps will help you to fulfill your greatest potential and find your purpose; your one ticket to living an amazing life – the incredible life that you are meant to live.

The combination of these steps will dramatically enhance the quality of your life by bringing you into harmony and alignment with the reason for your creation. This combination provides the answer to any search that you've ever had for meaning for your life. It is very possible to both make a living and create a life filled with abundant love, pleasure, happiness and meaning when you fulfill your absolute highest potential. Imagine a life where you can combine making a living with doing what you absolutely love every day. You'll discover the freedom that you've been craving so long and you'll awaken to what is truly most important in your life, rendering to the world your unique inner drive.

Once you discover your purpose you will find your life to be satisfying, joyous and highly fulfilling, even without making any external changes. You'll find that your health, energy levels, relationships and emotions will all improve as you align yourself with the nature of your life. Suddenly things will seem to make sense. As farfetched as this all may sound to you right now, you'll come to realise that nothing 'negative' or 'bad' can ever happen to you once you've aligned yourself with your purpose and that every single event that has ever happened in your life has shaped you into the person that you need to be so that you can fulfill your reason for living on this earth.

Above all else, within the significance of finding and fulfilling one's purpose lies the prime reason why everyone has been created with a specific purpose, which is to *give it to the world*.

This book isn't a quick fix; this is a blueprint that enables you to live a life of meaning and value, whilst at the same time helping you to give meaning to the lives of others. I'm going to dispel myths so that you can stop chasing what you *think* will make you happy, and give you the guidance needed to find what brings true happiness and well being.

By the time you've finished this book, you will know that you have the power, the strength and the courage to live life on your terms. No longer will you be trapped by mediocrity or be living a life that other people want you to live or a life that you think will please others. Instead, you will discover your infinite potential, be able to fully express the true you and have the choice and vigour to live the life that you want and need – the life worth living that you have previously been deprived of that you could have been living all along.

There is nothing more satisfying than finding and living your purpose. It's time for you to stop making excuses for why you aren't living the life you want and to begin fulfilling your destiny.

MY LIFE

I'll give you a quick overview of my life thus far so that you have an idea of how I got to the point where I'm now teaching others about living their purpose. To say that I've had an incredible journey over the past ten years is a massive understatement. I've been arrested, kicked out of school, money hungry, selfish, unhappy, anxious, fearful and insecure and then turned it all around to become a philosopher, life loving, meditating, spiritual, giving, caring, ultra happy human being. I've had many ups and downs and many slumps, but I would not change a single thing because I'm incredibly happy with where my life has progressed to. You'd be hard pressed to find a happier person living on this planet. I'm living my purpose, I love and am loved in return, and most importantly,

I use my passions, strengths and values every single day to help people live happier, more meaningful lives.

Going back five to ten years ago, I can see a dramatic shift in my persona. Back then, I grew up with fairly similar attitudes and values to those of my peers. I was always interested in what I could *get* from the world. I wanted money, properties, status and freedom — and lots of it. I constantly thought, 'What's in it for me?' and 'What can I get from this situation?' Like the majority of the people in this world, I was selfish and greedy and it seemed like nothing was ever good enough for me.

My poor attitude, insecurity and lack of values inevitably led me to being kicked out of my high school at the age of fourteen. My grades were terrible; I was hanging around the wrong crowd, smoking, drinking and fighting trying to acquire energy in all the wrong ways. Shortly after that I was arrested for stealing large amounts of money and stock from my part-time job. My poor parents had spent their entire lives doing all they could to provide the very best for me, and here I was throwing it right back in their faces. I was unappreciative and very badly behaved. They thought that I was washing my life down the drain and they didn't know how to control me. They tried everything they knew to change me but I simply wouldn't listen to them. As bad as I was, I'm willing to put myself in a vulnerable situation by telling you my life story and allowing you to know the person I truly was because I think it's very important for you to understand how this story links to my purpose. As bad as these times were for my parents, my family and myself, in hindsight I wouldn't change a thing because I know that everything that has happened in my life has helped me to grow into the person I am today.

Within the space of four years, a dramatic shift had started to form. My parents spent all their savings to send me to a great private school where I was surrounded by great people and mentors who helped me to develop a greater sense of integrity and responsibility. A few years later I was the School Captain, I completed my schooling with grades in the top 5% of Australia and I played football at the highest representative level for my age group. I got into my first preference for university and the future was looking bright. I'd made some remarkable life changes, had completely new values and was generally a completely new person.

But still, something was missing from my life. Do you know the feeling that I'm talking about — where everything seems fine from the outside, but still something is missing? Things seem to be going perfectly, you have the 'dream' job, the 'dream' partner or the 'dream' house, but you still feel empty. I felt that way for a few years. I was still focused on making money to the point where nothing was more important. I was constantly reading business books and searching for the next opportunity to make a big buck. I was still driven by greed and no matter what I had, I always wanted more. I'd study the world's greatest entrepreneurs and work out a plan to be just like them. Every cent that I earned was being gambled in the stock market into risky companies that I was sure were going to make me millions. I actually made quite a lot of money in the beginning, but inevitably, the millions never came and I gambled my life savings into evaporation. Something was missing for sure.

I began searching for more meaning in life. I thought, 'Surely there's more to life than the process of working hard in school so that I could get good grades that would eventually lead me to university, where I could work hard to get good grades so that I could get a good job, where I could work my butt off for forty years, sacrificing my happiness and spending restricted time with my family so that I could work my way up the corporate ladder so that I could one day retire rich.' I thought to myself, 'Really, what's the point of doing all that?' I decided right there and then that there is more to life and that I was not going to live a life of shallow existence, chasing empty goals like having more money, status, power and recognition. I realised that a life chasing those things is a life empty of meaning.

So I decided to dedicate *a lot* of my time into learning as much as I possibly could about personal development, happiness strategies, finding life's purpose and much, much more. I stopped working and began my quest for self-knowledge and wisdom. Along the way, I discovered some amazing people, authors, stories and learning tools that all taught me that *happiness, love* and *living a meaningful life* are so much more important than tangibles such as money, possessions or status. A few of them absolutely blew my mind and changed my life. As I began to embody what I was learning, my life was becoming happier and more joyous every day. In saying that, I'm not going to pretend like it was all smooth sailing; I still had certain things going on in my life that I had to conquer. Just because I was happy doesn't mean that my life was great all the time – I still had many fears to overcome – but my highs were consistently higher and my lows were much higher than they had been in the past. Without a doubt, the greatest investment you can ever make is that in yourself. Discovering who you truly are is far more valuable than anything else.

But still, I wasn't fulfilled. Something was still missing. There were still questions that I needed answers to. If one thing really leapt out at me, it was that **in order to live the most extraordinary, greatest life, one must combine their passions, strengths and values to provide a service to society**.

Everywhere I looked, all of the great philosophical teacher's seemed to say exactly the same thing; Martin Seligman, Wayne Dyer, Abraham Maslow, Deepak Chopra, Paulo Coelho, Marcus Aurelius, Ralph Waldo Emerson, Buddha, Socrates, Russell Simmons and many more all believe that we each have our own specific life purpose, and that our job is to find that purpose and then give it to the world. Let's be frank, these guys aren't exactly small-fry; they are some of the greatest thinkers and philosophers that the world has ever seen. I found that these scholars each believe that every living person has a purpose, and that one's purpose lies within one's passions, strengths and values. Furthermore, they believe that when one finds and fulfills their passions, strengths, and values, one is able to create a truly magical, happy and fulfilled life. I had a great epiphany when I learnt that we can all combine doing what we love, doing what we're great at, providing a meaningful service and making a living at the same time. This was a *big* realisation.

So off I set to find my passions, strengths and values. I wanted to discover exactly who I was so that I could fully give myself to the world. In doing so, I created a learning tool that you will find in this book to help you do exactly the same. A few months later, I'd discovered my passions, strengths and values, found my purpose, and found a way to make a living fulfilling my highest potential whilst also having a positive impact on the world. I realised that I loved learning about how to live my greatest life, I loved and was good at helping others, and I was tired of seeing so many people who felt unhappy and 'stuck' in their life situations. I had a strong desire to help others to live lives where they would be able to express their authentic selves and find an abundance of love, meaning and bliss. It was at that stage that everything that has ever happened in my life wonderfully started to feel connected. I finally found the meaning that was missing in my life for all those years, and was ready to fulfill my purpose, which I believe is to inspire many people to live happier, more loving and more fulfilled lives. Writing this book is the first step in my journey. I simply can't explain how much joy I get from using my passions and strengths every day in an effort to help people.

I tell you my story with the upmost humility. If the 'bad' things like getting arrested and kicked out of school had never happened, there is no way I would be the person that I am now.

If you're searching for deeper meaning in your life, this book will help you to find the answers that you need. Once you've read this book and completed all of the activities within, you will have discovered your truest self, your truest values, your greatest passions and strengths, your life's purpose and how you to get paid to do what you love. You'll then be in a position to fully express yourself to the world and live a life of deep meaning and connection to others.

Spirituality

There certainly aren't many more contentious questions to answer than 'Is there a God?' Before I begin to give you my thoughts on spirituality, know that when I discuss God/the Universe/the Creator/ Universal Energy/ the Divine/your Higher Power/whatever you want to call it, I'm not talking about any particular religion. I'm a very spiritual person yet I don't believe in a particular religion. I believe that most religions have some great philosophies and beliefs, but I'm unwilling to say that any religion is ultimately accurate. Regardless of your religious beliefs, all religions are about finding a relationship with a Higher Power. I do indeed believe that there's a Higher Power that created this world and I believe that same Power flows through each and every human, animal and plant in this world – I am just unwilling to categorize this Power and limit myself to the restrictions that most religions hold. Colloquially, the term 'God' has become misused, so I prefer to call this Higher Power 'Universal Energy'.

Even though my personal belief is that we have a reason to be here and a specific purpose for our lives, you are still free to make a choice, to exercise your Free Will, to choose, in the case of following my ideas and suggestions, to realise your potential and live a life of integrity and service or carry on living in an unfulfilled and selfish way.

When I was younger I travelled the world in search of what made some people successful and what held others back from achieving their greatest potential. Since my early teen years I've always been searching for what makes the difference between the great people who create tremendous change in this world and the 'Average Joe'. In search of this knowledge I travelled throughout the USA, Europe, Asia and Australia.

As my research has progressed, I've found the typical answers; hardwork ethic, natural talent, persistence, diligence, tenacity, passion, using one's strengths and following one's purpose – but everyone knows that these traits are vital, right? I needed to find more. On my quest I found two life changing pieces of wisdom. Firstly, all over the world I found that one trait stands out in nearly every human being. Everywhere I went, no matter what the culture or level of education, wealth or living standards, this same trait was evident in every area of my travels. I met and interacted with many lovely, caring people, but the trait that I speak of – *selfishness* – was evident in a large majority of the people that I saw.

The majority of people in this world dominantly value their own needs over the needs of others. Desperately wanting to know what caused this epidemic, I spent much time researching. I have since learned that the sole reason for selfishness is **lack of universal energy** – the one thing that determines the quality of our lives – in individuals and collective society. People are selfish because they are low on vital Energy.

Being low on Universal Energy is the number one cause of mediocrity and unfulfilled potential in all individuals and this in turn leads to selfishness.

With this knowledge, I am not surprised when I find that in conjunction with persistence and a hard work ethic, being spiritually connected and having a consistent stream of Universal Energy flowing through oneself is perhaps the most important condition you can attain if you wish to become extraordinary. Even though it's potentially the most important topic that one can even learn about, something has strangely kept spirituality and spiritual energy ignored in our society.

Now though, the rise of Eastern philosophies in the Western world is continually growing the sense that the spirit and soul is of greater importance that the physical self. The Being that is your soul holds much greater power and potential than the physical body and brain could ever muster. The world that we live in will feel a positive shift as its inhabitants begin to realise that each and every person is guided by a Universal Energy that we cannot tangibly see. Mankind have always exercised the body yet have neglected to exercise the most important part of their being, the energy of their spirit. It is essential that you become a spiritual person if you want to live an incredible life. Once you open yourself to the power of the universe, you will then be prepared to live the amazing life that you were truly meant to live. As you become spiritual you will notice a tremendous shift in your energy and your life will progress to a completely new level.

The people and associations that have made the greatest impact on this world have all been guided by a spiritual belief. Think of all the greatest teachers and doctrines – they have all been spiritual. These include the big religions such as Christianity, Buddhism, Judaism, Islam, Sufism and Confucianism plus numerous others, and people such as Mahatma Gandhi, Mohammed, Jesus Christ, Nelson Mandela, Ralph Waldo Emerson, Albert Einstein and many more. This list includes the greatest philosophers of past and present. It seems to me that the people who are having the greatest positive impact on our world in current times are also all connected spiritually and place a greater emphasis on their spiritual being than they do their physical being.

Think of the most influential teachers of our day; Deepak Chopra, Wayne Dyer, Oprah and Paulo Coelho among many others. All of these people are making an incredible impact in this world. The each do what they love, they each do what their good at and they each make a living fulfilling their purpose and helping the world – *they are all spiritual.* I have absolutely no doubt that the reason why these idols are having such a profound impact on society is because they all have a spiritual connection. Of course, success is not strictly limited to those spiritually inclined; you can certainly find influential atheists, although history shows that profoundly successful atheists are far less common. Wherever you look, if someone is having an enormously positive impact on the world and is living an incredible life, it is highly likely that this person is spiritually inclined.

You too have the power to be just like these heroes. Every human being is blessed with their own set of unique passions, strengths and skills which they are *made* to give the world.

If you want to live a blissful life, you must become a spiritual person and look to give your greatest passions, strengths and values in greatest service to the world.

Until you are able to find the spiritual essence of your being you will be continually focused on things which you think are important, but are not important at all. You will be focused on things *outside* of you as an approach to finding happiness and meaning. You will be focused on what you can acquire and how you look in the judgmental eyes of others. You will focus on having more and being more. That is why the world has become so materialistic and void of meaning. We have lost touch with our spirit.

It is now time to create a new world. Right now, the world places such a great emphasis on acquiring more; more money, more cars, more properties. People want to acquire more status, more power and they unconsciously chase these things thinking that they will find fulfillment. Yet love, happiness and meaning will never be found by accumulating 'more'. By trying to improve your status instead of looking to give your greatest passions and strengths in service to the world, you're switching off the bright light within you that is yearning to express your unique skills and individuality. You were born into this world with nothing material and you'll eventually leave this world with nothing material.

The question you must ask yourself is; **is there really any point in constantly trying to acquire more and 'be' more, if I'm eventually going to leave this world without all that I accumulate anyway?**

If you want to feel consistent happiness, meaning and love, you must know that you are not here to 'get', 'take' or 'have' – you are here to give. Humans don't exist to compete for who can acquire the most money or who can gain the most envy from others; humans are made to fulfill their purpose; to give, to love, to follow their hearts and to fully express their uniqueness.

LIFE'S GREATEST LESSON #1

Everything Is Connected

The most important discovery that you can ever have in your lifetime is to realize that there is a Higher Power that created and sustains this great world. It cannot be overstated just how much your life will be positively changed forever when you make this discovery. When you align yourself with Universal Energy you will begin to sustain the greatest feelings of inner peace, appreciation and happiness as you develop a new feel for the beauty and perfection of the world you live in. You'll realize that the happiness and meaning that you've always been searching for is already in your life everywhere you look and you'll begin to see the divine excellence in the things that you've previously taken for granted. You'll begin to find greater meaning behind everything in your life and discover that all aspects of this world are connected. Instead of simply seeing the world that surrounds you, you'll begin to feel perfect energy everywhere you go.

You have Free Will to exercise for the good of yourself and others, however, until you make this discovery the tremendous beauty that surrounds you will remain barely visible. You'll miss the perfect ambiance in every moment and will instead continue to chase things that will never give you the happiness that you're looking for. Everything will remain dull in comparison to the brightness of life that you will feel deeply when you become connected. You'll see glimpses once in a while, but you won't know the true beauty that life has to offer until you have aligned yourself with the Energy that created you as well as the world that you live in. When you realise that the same Energy that created this world also flows through you, you'll literally begin to feel amazed everywhere you go. You'll feel a deep sense of gratitude and appreciation for *everything* in your life. The deeply spiritual Mahatma Ghandi once said, "*When I admire the wonder of a sunset or the beauty of a full moon, my soul expands in worship of the Creator*". Ghandi understood the importance of aligning oneself with the divinity of life and used his connection to this Energy to fulfill his potential and create positive change in the world.

Every single thing that surrounds you has been purposely created by the same Energy. Take a look around you right now. What do you see? Wood, metal, concrete, materials, etc? They were all created purposefully by a Higher Power. The materials of the wooden chair you sit on, the clothes you wear, the car you drive, the concrete roads you drive on, the air you breathe, the bed you sleep on; the brain that you use to process this book, these have all been produced using resources that Universal Energy created. Realise that *everything* in this world has been purposely produced for the world's inhabitants.

If you're still not quite sure about the Energy of which I speak, I beg that you take a good look at the world around you. Surely you can't find it coincidental or by pure chance that we are such amazing beings in such an amazing world. Everything in this world is pure Intelligence.

Think about the human body and brain. It's estimated that the human body has ten trillion nerve cells which all have a specific purpose. Our brain has amazing functions. It's incredible how we can read these words and process the meaning behind them.

I can't remember the last time that I *consciously* digested my food, blinked to stop dust from getting into my eyes, made my heart beat, repaired my muscles and cells whilst I slept or made my fingernails grow. I can't remember the last time I consciously became attracted to someone of the opposite sex. I can't remember the last time I consciously cried when something sad happened. All of these things happen automatically without us even needing to think. Divine intelligence is driving our existence.

The human body is an incredibly created machine. It knows when to sleep, wake up, go to the bathroom; it even knows when to sweat to cool the body down and maintain the perfect temperature for the body to optimally function. It knows when to blink, how frequently to beat the heart and when to regenerate new cells.

Men and women are each designed differently and purposefully to carry out specific human functions. Our eyes are more precise than any camera that has ever been created; our ears can detect sound better than any piece of technology whilst at the same time providing us balance. Our digestive system takes all of the nutrients out of the foods we eat and discards the waste that the body doesn't need with superb ease.

How about the incredible reproductive system of life – a man and woman's reproductive organs fit perfectly to bring together a microscopic sperm and egg that grow into a full sized human. And above all else lays the incredibly organized structure of DNA – a nucleic acid that contains the genetic instructions used in the development and functioning of *all* known living organisms. It is very hard to believe that all of this is purely coincidental. Human life is simply too extraordinary to be anything other than divine. Surely there is a Creator and certainly this Creator didn't construct everything that lies in this astounding world for no good reason.

Think about the world that we live in. Do you really think that there is anything other than a Higher Energy that allows the sun to rise and set to change daytime into night time – every single day? It is beyond doubt that there is a Higher force of Energy that provides and sustains us with food grown from the ground and water from the sky. It is impractical to think that there is anything other than a Higher force that makes the leaves fall in the autumn and the flowers bloom in the spring. Surely there's a force that grows the grass, the roses and other beautiful plants in your garden. There must be a force that opens the petals of a flower during the day time so that it can gain energy from the sun, only to then close the petals when the sun goes down, day after day after day. Surely there's an energy that holds the planets in perfect orbit and keeps the moon in perfect lunar cycles. Surely there's a force that creates the perfect amount of gravity on planet earth so that nothing floats away.

The Earth is a perfect elliptical shape and is in a perfect position from the sun so that humans don't melt nor freeze. Earth contains the perfect concentrations of chemical that are needed to support all life and spins at a perfect rate that allows the cycle of the same seasons at the same time, year after year, century and century. We simply wouldn't survive if Earth was located anywhere else in the Milky Way.

The sun provides us with the most efficient form of energy needed to support life. The Earth is surrounded by an ozone layer that prevents lethal gases and ultraviolet radiations from affecting us, yet allows essential heat and light to reach us. Even the moon has the very important purpose of sustaining the ocean's tides and magnetizing the Earth so that it continues to spin stably on its axis. Without the moon, water would flood the Earth and life wouldn't exist.

On this Earth we are provided with the perfect level of oxygen to survive, and even that is incredible in itself. The Universal Power created an amazing process called photosynthesis whereby plants and trees transfer the carbon dioxide that we exhale into oxygen, creating a never ending supply. I'm discussing things on a very basic level here – the science behind all this stuff will blow your mind!

Even the animal kingdom and circle of life are amazing, unexplainable systems. Take close inspection to one of the 100 million different forms of species roaming this planet and you will find that each has an amazingly precise arrangement of parts. There's something incredibly perfect about our world and all of its inhabitants. We've been provided with an Earth that has everything we could even need not just to exist, but to prosper.

And as big as this Earth that we live on may seem, it is only a miniscule part of our galaxy, which is a minuscule fraction of what we know exists. Can all this be a coincidence? I think not. Everything is created for a specific reason. The complexity of the world goes far beyond chance and far beyond what the human mind can theorise. Do you really think that we have been solely created for anything other than a grand purpose?

There cannot be any doubt that the world is sustained by a much Higher Intelligence. The world and its inhabitants are too perfect to be anything other than divine. As a whole, we need to learn to trust in this Intelligence. We are all divine beings, we are all meant to be great and we are all connected by the same Energy force. Without doubt then, there must be a purpose for each and every human life.

We all have the extraordinary within us.

The same Energy that created this incredible world also created you. The entire world is pure intelligence, and it is up to us to recognise this and look for deeper meaning in our lives by discovering who we truly are and how we fit in to this great puzzle – to find our purpose – to be specific. We can learn so much from the beauty that surrounds us once we begin to align ourselves with it. When you know that the same Energy that created you also created this perfect world, you can trust that everything in your life is going to work out fine. If a Higher Power has the ability to create food, water and materials for specific purposes, you can rest assured that same Power has created a purpose and reason for your life. When you're spiritually disconnected from this source, it's likely that you'll live a life of constant frustration, unhappiness and continuous search for meaning. However, once you realise that you and *everything* else in this world was purposely created by a Higher Power, and then connect yourself to that Energy, you will begin to discover a life truly worth living.

SCEPTICISM

Before we go any further, I'd like to challenge any potential scepticism that you may have towards what this book discusses. Since I am discussing spirituality – a human impulse – I can understand if you are skeptical about what I'm talking about. Years ago, I too was skeptical about the notion of having a Higher Power and a purpose. I ask that you go beyond logic and try not to be skeptical. Approaching this topic with an open mind could well be the difference between living a life of suffering and living a life of extraordinary well being.

Our minds have been conditioned to 'believe what we can see' and unfortunately most people refuse to believe the things which they cannot understand. Before planes, microwaves, televisions and radios were invented, nobody could ever have imagined any of these technologies. 'Friends' of Guglielmo Marconi – the inventor of the radio – tried to put him in jail and labeled him insane when he told them about the possibility of hearing sound waves through a wooden box. Similarly, nobody believed there to be microscopic life before the microscope was invented. And who would have ever thought that we could search and find *anything* we wanted on a plastic screen via the internet?

Be willing to go beyond your rational mind and see that we are more than human bodies – we are souls and we are each meant to be. Closing your mind to such tremendous possibilities will stifle your creative imagination and hold you back from finding the meaning that you've always been searching for; keeping an open mind to the possibility of a Higher Power will allow you to find the great potential that lies dormant within you. You can't see oxygen, electricity, gravity, love or the bond that connects you to others, yet you know all of these exist.

At the time of writing, I estimate that very few people are aware that they have a purpose to fulfill during their life on Earth. Those who *are* aware are the people who are living peaceful, meaningful, loving, fulfilling, happy lives. These people realize that they have been born with unique gifts and are thus using them to make an impact in the world. They include the great teachers, artists, musicians, parents, leaders, physicians, and businesspeople. The goal of the book is to increase the number of people living purposefully. Imagine a world where every single person aligned with the purpose of their life. Imagine the incredible love and happiness between all humans and all of nature. Keeping an open mind to such an occurrence is the first step towards bringing this optimal world to life.

After reading this book, only those who *lack the courage* to follow their destiny and who can't see themselves living an incredible life will be the ones who are skeptical of its contents. Don't let the limitations that your ego creates stop you from living the life that you are *meant to live*.

The fact that you are already reading this book shows that you are in search of more meaning in your life. Be mindful of Universal Energy. You will find the signs all around you – in the grass that you walk on, the food that you eat, the oxygen you breathe, the warmth of the sun, the water you drink, the glory of nature, the clothes that you wear and every single item that is in your life. Embracing the unknown with trust and faith will allow you to create an incredible life.

Look for beauty all around you. Don't just look at objects; fully immerse yourself in their beauty. Appreciate yourself and your world as you realize that everything that surrounds you is divine beauty.

LIFE'S GREATEST LESSON #2

Everything Happens For a Reason

You will realise that nothing is anywhere as near as important as you've thought as you begin to move closer to knowing that there is a Higher Energy. Suddenly the things that currently cause you stress, fear, worry and anxiety will begin to lose their significance. It seems to me that humans take life way too seriously and place great emphasis on that which is not important. We're tightly wound and seem to get angry, annoyed and stressed at the smallest of issues. You will come to learn that everything happens for a reason and that there is no such thing as 'bad' or 'negative'. Just as a university leads its students towards finding a job, the school of life is not chaotic; rather, it provides learning to help you grow and fulfill your potential.

There is no such thing as a random event, there is no such thing as misfortune and there is certainly no such thing as bad luck. Nothing ever has or ever will occur in your life by chance or coincidence – everything that happens to you has meaning behind it and is leading you to where you need to be. Nothing will ever happen in your life that is not meant to happen because everything is always leading you towards fulfilling your purpose. Even within the most random and painful experiences lie the seedlings to a much larger, higher purpose. Everything that happens is *meant* to happen.

To create true greatness in your life, it's important that you shift your perspective from seeing yourself as a purely physical person with a body and mind, to being a spiritual person having a human experience, an energy field connected to the great Energy that created your life and world. You are more than just a human body living your life on earth; you are a soul with a connection to the Higher Intelligence that flows through you. Just as the world we live in is perfect intelligence, so too are you.

If it is difficult for you to see yourself as a spiritual person, try to consider yourself as part of the bigger picture. You are one of over six billion people who live on this purely divine earth. You are a tiny speck on this planet, which is a tiny speck of this galaxy, which is one tiny speck of the universe. There is a Higher Power that has created all this and that same power created and flows through you. The same power turns day into night and winter into spring. There simply are no accidents in this great world.

The idea of eternity will also help you to shift towards being a spiritual person. Eternity is a complex concept to try to get your mind around – like spirituality, it is a human impulse rather than a purely scientific fact. I'm simply asking you to keep an open mind on the idea. You know that the world was in existence for millions of years before your birth and that it will likely continue to be so for millions of years beyond your death. For all we know, the world has no beginning and no end – we can't prove either way.

Once you realize that all forms are impermanent, you can find peace by discovering and connecting with what is truly important – your eternal soul. Everything is unstable and will eventually perish. Beyond form, however, which is to say beyond anything physical, there is an aspect of you that survives and lives on beyond birth and death. As a collective society we've become so absorbed by making ourselves look better that we're neglecting our eternal essence. People are willing to spend vast amounts of money and time making their bodies look better through going to the gym, eating healthy foods, applying make-up and looking fashionable, yet are unwilling to look beyond that captivation to discover their essence; the part of them that goes beyond materialism, form and content. Beyond the content of our lives lays something much more important. Each human being is a soul of divine origin, yet each human being is focusing too much energy on that which is not important, including forms and content, to the point where we've forgotten that origin, which is our eternal soul. The form identity that the ego tries to emphasize as being most important pales in significance compared to your true origin.

Have you ever questioned why one day you came from nothingness to somethingness? On the day of your birth you came from no form to form. Why do you think it is that you are born into this great world, only to die a certain number of years later even though the world continues to go on normally? Have you ever consciously reflected on your unique place in the scheme of human evolution? I propose that there is a reason – a Grand Mission – firstly that defines why you were born and secondly that defines why you were born on the specific date that you were. There is a reason why you went from nothingness to human existence. You are here to accomplish your grand purpose and every moment of your life has led you to where you are now and will continue leading you until you fulfill your purpose. Each and every person has their own specific purpose or mission on this earth and this book has been created to help you find yours. To find and live your purpose, you first have to realize that you are a spiritual being. If the universe can keep the seasons changing, the planets turning perfectly and create something as divinely beautiful as the human being, rest assured that it's going to have plans for you! So allow the Energy to flow through you, look for and feel the beauty that surrounds you and find the brilliance in every single life form in this amazing world.

With this in mind, think back over your life and contemplate how every event has led you to the next, and so on, until you find yourself here today. Just as I discussed with my journey, every single event that has happened in your life has led you to where you are today. If you look back over your life you'll see that *everything* has happened in your life for a reason. Everything that has happened in your life has been preparing you all along for your purpose. Your life is one big story in your search for your purpose. Though you may not have realized this; this book can help you uncover that purpose.

When I look back, it's crystal clear to me. Upon reminiscence of my childhood, I have constant memories of people close to me complaining about their jobs. One can sense the energy that those who are not fulfilling their potential carry within them, and I could certainly feel that energy emanating from many of the people that I came into contact with when I was younger. Lacking the courage to follow their hearts and fulfill their potential, these people would show up tightly wound and stressed day in and day out, constantly complaining about their situation and then finding a way to numb their existence. At the time this really angered me. I noticed that many of the people close to me were never present in their roles as parents, friends and partners because they were too consumed in the problems of their own life. I thought to myself, 'Why would people continue with the same job day in and day out, year after year, when they didn't even like the job, when it so evidently sucked their energy dry?' I simply could not make any sense of people choosing to live like this. As I became aware of this, I noticed more and more people whose jobs hindered, rather than supplemented their lives.

Now when I look back I can see that this situation was absolutely perfect because it enforced a drive inside of me to want to help people follow their passions and purpose and love their work – which is exactly what I'm doing now. As I continually noticed people suffering from not fulfilling their highest potential, I realized that things needed to change. I hated seeing those close to me so visibly upset all the time, to the point that it has engrained a tremendous drive in me to help prevent others from being in that situation. Thus, I can see greater meaning and reasoning behind a previously 'negative' situation.

What Changed Me

Along the way, I dabbled in the share market and made quite a lot of money, which led me to believe that I could be a full time investor. At this point, I became really greedy. I wanted more money and I wanted it quickly. When I became a full-time investor, it seemed that it didn't matter where or what I invested in, I always lost money – and lots of it. It sucked. At the time I was as money hungry as they come. It definitely hurt to see so much money being lost at the time, but now I can look back and see how perfect that this time of my life was, that it was not accidental and that it led me towards finding my purpose. If I'd continued to make money, I would still be chasing the next big investment to this very day. Instead, I was turned off from investing which lead me in a new direction toward doing what I do now.

When I was younger I got kicked out of school. I lost friends, divided my family and embarrassed my parents. It was one of the worst periods of my adolescence, but now when I look back I can see that negative event led me to finding the love of my life and future wife at my new school, becoming school captain and gaining some extraordinary education which I would not have had at my previous school.

When I was fifteen I was arrested and fired for stealing from my employer. I caused my parents grief beyond belief, was grounded for a *long* time and had all of my privileges taken away from me. I was also publicly shamed. That was also a really bad period of my life; however, looking back I can see how that period strongly influenced me in becoming extremely self-disciplined and to living my highest level of integrity.

At the age of twenty two I became severely sick when travelling solo through India. I was in such intense pain that I was unable to leave my bed and had no support. It was a really tough experience that pushed my comfort zone beyond belief. At the time, it was probably the 'worst' experience of my life. Yet, when I look back now I can see that it really helped me to grow as a person. The situation helped me to become much more independent and also to increase my empathy towards others who suffer.

These are the bigger episodes of my life, but literally something happens every day to teach me what I need to learn to grow. If none of these things had happened, I wouldn't be the person that I am now. All that I needed to learn and grow came to me at the precise right moment. I certainly haven't got everything that I've ever wanted from life, but I've got no doubt that I've always received what I've needed to fulfill my potential.

Looking back over my life, I can honestly say that nothing 'bad' or 'negative' has ever happened to me and that every failure or 'bad' period throughout my life brought with it a great lesson and the seed of an equivalent success. To paraphrase Buddha, every event that ever happens in your life is empty of meaning other than the meaning which you give it. If you say that something is 'good', then it's good. If you say that something is 'bad', then it's bad, but ultimately, everything is empty. There is no such thing as 'good' or 'bad', everything simply *is* – everything has a higher order and purpose. It simply comes down to the perspective or meaning that you place on it. So when you can grasp the empowering spiritual perspective that 'everything happens for a reason', even when something 'not so great' happens in your life, you realize that the event has greater meaning behind it and is, in fact, helping you to grow towards your potential. I'm delighted that all of the 'bad' things happened to me because they allowed me to grow into the person who I am now – and I love that person.

Life will always give you what you need, when you need it. Steve Jobs once spoke about how we must trust that everything is happening for a grand reason. Jobs said, *"You can't connect the dots looking forward. You can only connect them looking backwards, so you have to trust that the dots will somehow connect in your future. You have to trust in something — your gut, destiny, life, karma, whatever — because believing that the dots will connect down the road will give you the confidence to follow your heart, even when it leads you off the well-worn path, and that will make all the difference."*

Throughout all of my 'troubled' times I could never see the grander picture. I was stuck in the moment and could not connect the dots looking forward. Nowadays, I can look back and see how the dots have always connected perfectly at the exact precise moment. With such great knowledge from my experiences, I now have confidence and trust throughout the times of uncertainty and know that everything will eventually connect, no matter how uncomfortable the situation is in the present moment. This allows me to follow my heart, even when it leads me off the well-worn path.

Many of the world's most successful people also realize that *everything happens for a reason*, and have lived their life accordingly. Possibly the greatest example can be found within the life of Oprah Winfrey. Oprah experienced a childhood of much adversity to say the least. Oprah was raped, sexually abused and lived in a very poor family. However, Oprah overcame such adversity to become one of the world's most admired women by using the intense emotions that she felt inside her to motivate and empower millions of people all over the world. She once said, *"We all stumble. We all have setbacks. If things go wrong, you hit a dead end — as you will — it's just life's way of saying time to change course. ... If you really get the lesson, you pass and you don't have to repeat the class. If you don't get the lesson, it shows up wearing another pair of pants — or skirt — to give you some remedial work."*

Rather than using her life circumstances as an excuse or reason to hold her back, Oprah embraced her 'negative experiences' and used her past to create greatness in her life and the lives of many others.

Likewise, Steve Jobs, the creator of Apple and one of the world's greatest businessmen, also endured many struggles along his journey. Jobs was fired by Apple — the very company that he created — many years ago. During his time away from Apple, Jobs became the CEO of Pixar Animations and founded Next Computers. These great companies would never have existed if he didn't get fired from Apple. At another point in his life, Jobs was told that he had a lethal cancerous tumor in his pancreas. With the thought that he was going to die, Jobs began living his life as if every day was his last. After later finding out that his tumor had been cured, Jobs said, *"Almost everything — all external expectations, all pride, all fear of embarrassment or failure – these things just fall away in the face of death, leaving only what is truly important. Remembering that you are going to die is the best way I know to avoid the trap of thinking you have something to lose. You are already naked. There is no reason not to follow your heart."*

Rather than feeling sorry for himself, Jobs discovered that *everything happens for a reason*, and from that time on, lived his life to its fullest potentialities.

These are just some of the examples of great people who have not only overcome their 'problems', but have used them to benefit their lives as well as the lives of others. In fact, it seems (although not always the case) that the people who go through the most pain, whether that be sexual abuse or physical or psychological pain, are often the people who contribute the most to society and make the most positive changes in the world. These people don't sulk, they don't complain and they certainly don't use these 'bad' moments to make excuses for why they can't fully express themselves. Instead, they take strength from their situations and realize that when one door closes, another door opens. They don't see their problems as the 'end of their world' – they view them as an opportunity in disguise – *a new beginning*. They see these moments as an opening of higher order and a turning points towards their new lives.

Similarly to myself and others described, you too can draw from your past and see how the dots have connected for you. Think back over your lifetime and discover how every 'bad' event that has ever happened in your life has led you to who you are now. Once you believe in this and see every event in your life as a privilege, an opportunity to grow and an improvement in your character, you'll open yourself up to receiving increased assistance from Universal Energy, you will start getting more support in your endeavors and will sense greater meaning behind every event in your life, even the mundane.

Think about anything 'bad' that has happened in your life. Bad break-ups, illnesses, deaths, depressions, addictions, job loss...anything 'bad' that you're holding onto. If you look back you'll discover that every event that has happened in your life was necessary to bring you to where you are now, even if you didn't understand the greater meaning behind the event at the time that it occurred. Every single event that ever has and ever will happen in your life has a *purpose*. Knowing this, if anything ever goes not according to the way you plan or hope, you can always find answers within, and these answers unlock knowledge that you *need* to discover. Misfortune, temporary defeat, pleasure and pain all teach us incredible lessons and provide us with inner growth that we *need* to fulfill our reason for existence.

Many people hold on to pain from their childhoods. If this is the case for you, you're definitely not alone. Go back to your childhood and think about anything that you may be holding onto. Knowing that there is a reason for every single event and circumstance in your life – including the parents that you were born to – ask yourself either verbally or by writing in a journal:

- 'Why was I born to my particular parents?'
- 'What might be the higher purpose behind the things that I still hold onto from my childhood?'
- 'What would I change about my parents and my upbringing? What can I learn from these things?'

The final question, 'What would I change about my parents?' is vitally important for you to answer. In your answer lies an important *part of your purpose*. There is a reason why you were born to your parents, a reason why you endured their values and a reason why you were the recipient of the lessons that they taught you. It is imperative that you embrace this fact and understand that everything that has led you to be the person who you are right now is all *purposeful*. In fact, every event that ever happens in your life is positive, because behind each event lies an answer that is helping you to evolve into the person that you are *meant* to be so that you may live the life that you are meant to live.

All of your problems and the things that you hold onto from the past will be 'cleared' when you acknowledge that *everything happens for a reason*. It's likely that you've gone through suffering during your lifetime, but with hindsight, you can realise that you've grown and learnt through every experience that you've ever had – you can connect the dots.

If there are people in your life that you dislike, or you're unhappy with your childhood or they way that you parents treated you, know that every single person and circumstance that has even been and ever will be has a reason behind it. Trust that the universe has plans for you that go beyond what the mind can comprehend. Anything that ever happens in your life is always leading you toward your grand mission. Search for the significance, the message and the meaning behind everything that ever happens. Universal Energy has determined your destiny and your whole life is always directing you towards its fulfillment.

Many of us never realise this perspective and go through their entire life saying 'Why me?' and suffering. A very close person in my life held onto so much pain from her childhood that it completely affected her entire life. Her pain from the past literally affected her life to the point that she suffered in a way that you never want to see anyone suffer. She gave so much energy and resistance to her pain that it grew to the point that her only outlet was to consume herself in her job, which of course only created greater pain as the original cause of her pain was neglected. Her incessant thoughts and toxic energy towards the past stopped her from being in the present moment, which affected all of her relationships.

Rather than accepting whatever happens and searching for greater meaning, many of us form a barrier of resistance and let the past *control* our lives. Sometimes we can't clearly understand that things happen in our lives to help us learn and grow, thus as we fight what is, we inevitably feel anger, stress and resentment towards ourselves and others. Life will continue to repeat circumstances that make us feel uncomfortable until we learn the lesson that it is trying to teach us. If we don't learn from the lessons of our circumstances, our emotions will intensify to the point that we must give it our attention.

True happiness is never attainable for the person who cannot integrate their past into their present and leave the future clear. You only punish yourself when you hold on to anger and resentment over things from the past. The events of the past are gone, they're done and they will only continue to affect you based on the energy that you give them. Whether you give the events from your past positive or negative energy is completely within your control. You can't change what has happened in your life, so stop letting it affect you. Instead, see the greater meaning behind it. Those who constantly resist or fight against the complex forces that are creating their destiny and cannot realize that the conspiracy of coincidences that occur in their lives are what they *need* will inevitably suffer. Yet if these people searched for meaning behind these events, they would discover the great benefits and answers that Universal Energy has been trying to teach them. If you realise that you have the capacity to choose your response and find meaning behind the events in your life, you will grow exponentially.

All of the events that have happened throughout your lifetime have been leading you towards your purpose. Those who have the knowledge that everything is necessary understand that there simply are no accidents and that everything happens for a grand reason. They interpret such situations as being great gifts that allow them to grow. Instead of being the victim and asking 'Why me, God?', they live their lives feeling empowered that they are the creators of their circumstances and aren't the victims of what others do or don't do. Instead of thinking 'Why is this happening to me' they think 'This is what I need' and 'There is greater meaning behind this situation'. Simply, these people find the silver lining and meaning behind their life experiences, even when things aren't going to plan.

In every single moment of your life you have the choice to be either a creator or a victim of your circumstances. The easiest thing is to become entranced by the ego; the fear based part of your mind, and feel like the victim. The people who live the most fulfilling lives, however, do what others are unwilling to do; empower themselves by becoming the creator of their circumstances.

You have the power to choose the meaning that you place on any event. You always have the choice to decide whether to see the events of your life as a gift and opportunity to grow or as something that you will stop you from growing. Your life will be significantly different depending on whether you choose to be the creator or the victim.

Once you integrate the spiritual realization that everything happens for a reason, the next goal is to bring yourself to the point where you can see the answers as they come, rather than in retrospect. Forming this mental position will allow you to bring yourself to the point where you can see the answers as they happen in the moment. When you get to this point, you'll begin to question 'Why is this happening?', 'What can this teach me?', 'How can I grow from this experience?', and 'What do I need to change?' – even if whatever's happening feels negative at the time. You will learn, grow and improve with every single event and experience that you encounter in your life. If you want to follow your heart, express your true self and have confidence and trust throughout times of uncertainty with the knowledge that everything will eventually connect – no matter how uncomfortable the situation is in the present moment – you must learn to trust that everything happens in your life for a grand reason.

With this in mind, think back over your past experiences of pain, failure or defeat. What can you take or gain from what you've previously viewed as 'bad' situations? Within each painful experience lies a lesson that will help you evolve to bring you closer to your purpose. Never regret your past – it is your greatest teacher.

Begin at once to realize the great lessons that can be found in the pain that you still hold onto. Think about the things that you have learnt through these experiences. Each of these experiences have been leading you to the answers that you must find in order to live a purposeful life. The lessons hidden within the experiences that you have endured throughout your lifetime have always been leading you towards your purpose. And what about your current situation – are you having difficulties with your friends or family? Are people at work making you angry? Is your boss treating you like trash? Is your work stressing you?

Search for deeper meaning and find the lessons behind any 'problems' or 'bad' situations in your life – they hold the key to your destiny. Search for the hidden gifts that adversity is *giving* you so that you may create a more empowering understanding of your situations.

We need to step out of our situation and view everything that happens in our lives not through our instinctive emotions, but through the knowledge that every circumstance, event and person is connected to the whole. If we replace our emotions and thoughts with a spiritual view, we can see how everything has always been connecting us to our purpose and helping us to grow so that we may fulfill our very highest potential.

Your ability to fulfill your potential is determined by your perception and response to the challenges that life provides you along the way, and the growth and quality of your life is established by the way you respond to such challenges.

Life happens and you get to decide what every event means. In deciding that every event is leading you to living your highest potential, you create bliss beyond measure.

Empower yourself with the knowledge that *everything happens for a reason.* **Everything has a purpose!** Your life is unfolding *exactly* as it should.

Everything happens exactly as it's meant to happen. Behind everything lies hidden meaning.

Anything in your life that is 'bad' is exactly what you need right now in order to grow. When you begin to apply this perspective to every event in your life you will automatically feel less pain and much more meaning. You can begin to enjoy your days knowing that everything that happens in your life doesn't happen *to you*, it happens *for you*. Whatever happens, know that the whole universe is conspiring in your favor.

Never judge anything, simply accept everything. Everything is. Bring yourself to the point where you don't mind whatever happens. Regardless of what has happened, your resistance to what is cannot change what is. We have no power over the waves that roll in, however we can certainly learn how to ride then. Align yourself with Universal Intelligence and find greater meaning in every event. Consider everything that happens in your life as a gift from your Higher Power. *Everything in life is in perfect order*. Even this book has come to you because it is exactly what you *need* right now to help you evolve closer towards your purpose. Follow it, flow with what life has to offer you, and most importantly, don't miss the answers that life provides you.

CHAPTER SUMMARY

- Everything is always leading you towards where you need to be. Every event, situation and circumstance is purposeful and holds hidden meaning. True happiness is only attainable to those who can see this meaning.

- Life will always give you what you need, when you need it. All that you *need* to learn and grow always comes to you at the precise right moment. If you miss the lesson behind the events and circumstances that you are gifted with, the events will intensify, often to the point that you suffer until you learn the lesson. Any perceived problem that you have will vanish when you see the 'problem' for what it is – a gift that allows you to grow.

- You have the power to choose how you view and respond to all situations and events. To view all events as happening for a reason is to empower yourself, whereas to view events as 'negative' is to victimise yourself.

- If you want to follow your heart, express your true self and have confidence and trust throughout times of uncertainty with the knowledge that everything will eventually connect – no matter how uncomfortable the situation is in the present moment – you must learn to trust that everything happens in your life for a grand reason. You must trust that the dots will eventually connect.

PRACTICE

Think back over your life and discover how everything has always been leading you to being the person that you are now. Search for meaning behind past situations and events, especially those that you still hold on to. Shift your perspective so that you may learn the lesson that these events were trying to teach you. To resist the past is to suffer, whilst to embrace the past is to grow.

Search for meaning in everything that happens to you – even the most mundane events. Whenever an unfavourable event occurs, ask yourself, 'Why is this happening?', 'What can this teach me?', 'How can I grow from this experience?', and 'What do I need to change?' Constantly remind yourself that every event, circumstance and situation holds a lesson for you to seize.

Accept everything that happens to you with the knowledge that the world is in perfect order and that everything is *meant* to happen to you.

Remove the words 'negative', 'bad' and 'unfortunate' from your vocabulary – there is no such thing. Every event, situation and circumstance happens to allow you to grow.

LIFE'S GREATEST LESSON #3

Everything Has a Purpose

There are two great days in life – the day you are born and the day you discover why. You have been uniquely created and given specific gifts so that you are exceptionally brilliant at a certain thing – your purpose. Therein, you cannot be replaced – no matter how highly or lowly you regard yourself – you have been divinely created to be great at a specific vocation and the world needs you.

Your one and only central need in your life is to fulfill your own potentialities and use the gifts that you've been blessed with to give your greatest self to the world. You must trust that your guiding inner spirit/ Higher Power/God/Universal Energy is always guiding you throughout your life in order to help you fulfill your purpose. You *will* live a fulfilling and meaningful life once you begin to express your deepest inner drive and potentialities and follow your purpose. Conversely, if you live your life disregarding your unique gifts you will have betrayed yourself and your community and will thus suffer from adverse aspects. Take this literally. The cause of any adverse aspects in your life spurs from neglecting to express your inner power.

Everything is created for a purpose, from the computer or the paper that you're reading this from, to the water that you drink, to the chair that you sit in. The sun, moon, every single animal, plant, tree and fruit have all been created for a specific purpose. *Everything*. And so are all human beings. Everything in this world does what it's meant to do. A light globe fills a room with light, the sun warms the earth, fruit and vegetables provide the energy that we need through fibre, minerals and vitamins – everything in this world fulfills its purpose – humans need to learn to do the same. We're not just born onto this earth 'because' or by pure chance. We have each been uniquely created to fulfill a certain mission or purpose in life. Everything in this world is perfect Intelligence.

I implore you to consciously reflect on your unique place in the scheme of human evolution.

Think about how large the world is. Take a wander outside and look up at the stars one night and realise how small you are in comparison to your surrounds. You are just one tiny spec of a massively intelligent system. The world which we live in is incredibly large and every single organism has a specific purpose. Did you know that rainforests create fires every few hundred years to help the regrowth process? You would certainly have seen how leaves fall off trees in autumn and regrow to bloom in spring.

Just as there is a higher force that keeps the planets turning in perfect order and makes the flowers bloom in the spring, there is an intelligent force running through you. You have been put on this earth for a reason. You were born into this world to fulfill a grand mission. There is no such thing as pure chance. If Universal Intelligence can give a plant the required nutrients, soil, sun and water to grow healthily, have faith that if you align yourself with this power that everything that you need will also be provided to you.

So how do you know what your purpose is? And how do you find your purpose? Your purpose lies within discovering who you truly are, and most notably, discovering your passions, strengths and values. These qualities were given to you for a reason. In fact, all features and characteristics that you possess (no matter if you believe them to be good or bad traits) have been bestowed upon you as part of what you are meant to fulfill during your lifetime. Once you become spiritually connected to Energy, the next step is to discover your true self and find your greatest passions, strengths and values, and then work towards finding your purpose and bringing it to life. We each have extraordinary potential if only we would allow ourselves to search for it. It is your birthright to live a life of happiness, love and meaning and these will all come as a result of fulfilling your purpose.

Dreams and Desires

Any dream or desire that you ever have originates from Universal Energy. At a subconscious level, any desire that you have is given to you by your Higher Power as a means of expressing itself through you. Your desires are aligned with your strengths, passions, values and purpose. Everything is related, and just as everything happens for a reason, any desire that you have is given to you because Universal Energy is trying to express itself through you. The Energy wants you to fulfill your purpose and thus gives you the desire to do so. I'm not talking about sexual desires or desires of things that you think you 'should' have because you want to impress others, I'm talking about your deepest dreams and the things that fill you with excitement and enthusiasm when you think about them. Your deepest dreams and desires are highly correlated with your purpose.

I'm here to tell you that you can achieve any desire that you have. After all, the power that's given you the desire originally also has the power to make your desire come to life.

A desire is energy of thought which originates from the same energy that created this world and all of its inhabitants, including you. You need to believe that you can have *anything* that you desire and that anything that you want is achievable because your desires originate from Universal Energy. If this wasn't the case, you would not be given your desires in the first place. Once you believe that the same Energy that gave you your desires can also help you to bring them to fruition, your faith will allow you to see that if you follow your greatest desires, everything and anything is achievable and any anxiety and worry that you currently hold toward the future will dissolve because you'll know that any impulses that you have are Energy's means of expressing itself through you.

When you have a dream or desire, Universal Energy is trying to express itself through you and help you to give your purpose to the world. Your Higher Power wants you to give your unique strengths and passions to fulfill your reason for being here. Everything happens for a reason and everything has a purpose, including your thoughts and desires. The embodiment of this knowledge is vitally important.

At the level of form, all things that enhance our lives right now – aeroplanes, telephones, computers, the internet, and constructions – are the results of people who had the courage to fulfill their deepest desires. At the deeper level beyond form, the religions that empower billions of people throughout the world are also the result of those few people who followed the call of their deepest desires. You too can certainly create anything that you ever want – especially your deepest desires – when you connect with the same Energy that created our world, our galaxy, our earth and your personnel human self. When you do, you will most certainly create things that will enhance the lives of others.

Many people don't have the faith or trust that their desires are purposeful, and unfortunately push them aside because they either don't believe that they can achieve them or they lack the courage to try. Sadly, most of us are conditioned to chase for instant results, and if we don't get those instant results, we inevitably neglect our deepest desires and give up. It's not our fault – we're conditioned to be this way. We're surrounded by commercials, TV shows and movies where people reach their dreams with minimal effort. We see the commercials with models that have incredible bodies. We see the sports stars that are incredibly fit and mentally tough. We see the singer who can wow a crowd with seemingly minimal effort, we see the rich businessman living a life of luxury on his 100ft yacht. When we see these people and the lives they live we think, 'I want to be like that person'.

But what the TV shows, commercials, movies and successful people don't usually show us is the years of blood, sweat and tears that went into creating this greatness. We don't see the years of dieting and hard work that the models have put in at the gym, we don't see the long hours of practice that the sportspeople have put in for years on end, we don't see the endless hours that the businessman has spent working tirelessly and sacrificing his personal time with friends and family to make his fortune.

We're conditioned to think that we should get results *straight* away, and unfortunately we tend to quit when this inevitably doesn't happen. Come on! Everybody knows that nothing great is ever created overnight. So stop trying to gain instant rewards from minimal work. This meaningless existence is not good for your soul. Stop playing the lotto in search of the millions, stop playing the share market in search of the next big win and stop giving up at the first sign of failure. Instead, make an effort to learn who you truly are – I'm not talking about the person who society wants you to be – I'm talking about your truest essence.

When you've been given a desire – something that flows tremendous amounts of enthusiastic energy through your body – you must be willing to put in the energy and hard work to express them. Don't worry about how you will fulfill your desire or purpose; just know that you are capable, that you have a Higher assistance and that the answers you need will eventually come to you. Have faith that results will eventually come your way if you put in the required effort. Your Higher Power gives you your desires for a reason – it wants you to act on them so that it can fully express your greatest self within this world. If you lack the courage to fulfill your desire, it will eat away at your soul, which is what always happens when you don't fulfill your potential and don't act on the deep drive that you feel within; this is the prime reason that so many people search for an escape through excessive consumption of alcohol, drugs, sex and over eating. The majority of all of the problems in this world stem from people not having the courage to act upon their deepest drive. Every blessing ignored eventually becomes a curse. You must be willing to put in the work – and that starts with doing the questions in the later chapters of this book. The goal of this book is to move your desires from idle wishes and hopes to true expression of your highest self.

Enthusiasm

As you begin to find your purpose you will be filled with high levels of enthusiasm. Enthusiasm creates a clear path for creative manifestation. When you've found your purpose you will be awakened, full of enthusiasm, full of deep enjoyment and committed to achieving an incredible goal.

Enthusiasm is strongly aligned with your spirituality, your desires and your purpose. Did you know that enthusiasm translates from ancient Greek to mean 'God within' and 'to be possessed by a god?' Enthusiasm and passion are the two greatest energies that will ever flow through you, and they both originate from and connect you to Universal Energy. When you feel sustained levels of enthusiasm you have unlimited creative power flowing through your being because of the strong connection that aligns you with Energy.

Nothing great has ever been achieved without enthusiasm. Think about some of the most amazing man-made wonders of the world. One could stare at the Taj Mahal, the ancient Egyptian pyramids and Machu Pichu for hours and wonder how something so remarkable was ever created. Each of these man-made wonders was created hundreds, if not thousands of years ago. None of these would exist, had it not been for the enthusiasm and passion of their creators. Even cars, planes and motor vehicles would have seemed impossible to create right up until the moment that their enthusiastically connected creators brought them to life through expressing what was burning inside them.

When you are feeling enthusiastic, Universal Energy is flowing through you – literally. Not feeling enthusiastic or feeling anything other than passion and enthusiasm flowing through your body is a sure sign that you are not connected to your Higher Power – this is a great alarm clock trying to wake you up and tell you to become connected!

It is so important that you follow and connect with your desires, passions and whatever else makes you enthusiastic. To live an extraordinary life, you simply must love what you do. If you spend your life doing something that doesn't fire you up and flow enthusiasm through you, you'll spend your time going through the motions, never loving what you do, never doing your best, never fulfilling your potentialities and never living your most optimal life. As discussed earlier, if you want to fulfill your desires and become successful, you must be willing to put in the work. If you're enthusiastic about what you're working towards, you'll breeze through it. On the other hand, if you don't get enthusiastic or excited about your work, you'll lose interest, deliver low quality work and eventually end up quitting. This is why I keep stressing how important it is that you discover you passions and strengths and then give them to the world.

Here's some simple math. Enthusiasm + desire = connection with Universal Energy, creative power, intensity, enjoyment and bliss. If you want to live a fulfilled life, always listen to the call of your soul and look to energise yourself by doing that which makes you excited and enthusiastic.

CHAPTER SUMMARY

- Everything that you can see, feel, smell, touch, taste and hear has a purpose. Everything in this world fulfills the potentialities that it was created for.

- You have been uniquely created to fulfill a specific purpose. Everything that has ever happened in your life has been leading you towards a purpose that only you can discover and fulfill. This is the reason for your life on Earth.

- It is your birthright to live a life of happiness, love, meaning and fulfillment. All of these *will* come to you when you fulfill your potentialities and follow your purpose.

- To find your purpose you must discover your true self – most importantly, your passions, strengths and values.

- Your deepest desires are a gift from Universal Energy. The same Energy that gives you your desires also provides you with the means for fulfilling them. Universal Energy gives you your desires so that it may express itself though you and help you to give your purpose to the world.

- Your deepest desires are purposeful – you must take action to fully give yourself to the world in order to live a fulfilling existence.

- Enthusiasm is one of the greatest energies that will ever flow through you. If you want to live a fulfilled life, always look to energise yourself by doing things which you know fill you with excitement and enthusiasm.

PRACTICE

- Look for the purpose that lies within everything that surrounds you. Appreciate the beauty and perfection of all that you can sense, especially the beauty and perfection of yourself and the world that you live in.

- Take a moment to think about your deepest desires. Realise that your desires are a gift. What is holding you back from fulfilling your desires?

- Think about what gets you enthusiastic. How can you implement these things into your life more frequently?

LIFE'S GREATEST GIFT – UNIVERSAL ENERGY

Every single living creature requires Universal Energy to flow through them to maintain their existence here on earth. We all rely on this energy – it is what keeps us alive. After all, death is the ultimate loss of energy and when you die your universal and eternal energy moves into another form, continuing your soul's eternal life. Your body stays here on Earth and slowly decays into dust because it no longer holds the required energy to keep it vital. Whilst here on earth, the level of Universal Energy that flows through your body, mind and soul determines all of your actions and your quality of life. This is big. This connection to Energy is responsible for the way the world is right now, the way that you behave and the way that all of those around you behave.

This Universal Energy that I speak of is more powerful than anything else in this world. It originates and flows from the Creator of this world into every living thing. Everything in this world is made up of energy and matter. Take a look around you. What can you see? Whatever you're looking at is a vibrating Universal Energy field. **Everything that you see is vibrating energy**. Plants, animals, humans, your thoughts and the things that you perceive as hard matter such as the clothes you wear, the bed you sleep in, the chair that you sit on, your cell phone, the glass you drink from – whilst these things appear to be hard objects, they are all made up of energy that is vibrating at different frequencies.

Everything that you can sense with touch, sight, taste, sound and smell is vibrating energy. Every single object that you can sense, including this book that you are holding in your hands, is made of molecules, which are made of atoms, which are made of electrons, neutrons and protons, all of which are vibrating energy that is beyond the comprehension of the five human senses. What humans can physically sense is only a small fragment of the vibrational energy that surround us.

All energy is the same, only differentiated by frequency and intensity of vibration. All objects seem solid to the human eye, yet they are made of energy vibrating at different frequencies. Everything is alive! For example, the chair that you can see is made of the same energy as the book that you're holding and your human body itself, only they all differ in their frequency of vibration. Although your eyes can't sense it, the structure of the chair is not actually a solid object; it is empty space that is filled with lively, vibrating energy. The harder an object is, the slower its vibrational energy, and the softer an object is, the faster it's vibrational energy. For example, the energy that creates steel is the same energy that creates cotton, only the energy of steel vibrates at a much slower rate. Steel and cotton both appear to be solid to the naked human eye, yet at a deeper level they are made up of lively, intensely vibrating energy.

Everything in this world is made of energy, including heat, oxygen, sounds, light and water, the energy that makes up anywhere from 60-70% of the human bodies energy. Just as ice, water and steam are all the same energy only differing in their intensity of vibration, so is everything else that you can physically sense. Where does this energy originate from? It is Universal Energy, the same force that created and sustains this great world.

What our senses distinguish to be hard matter is really just empty space with intense energy flowing through it – and this includes the human body. The body is made up of trillions of cells, which like everything else in this world are made of molecules, which are made of atoms, which are made of electrons, neutrons and protons, all of which are vibrating energy. Every cell in the human body is an electric energy field. No matter your body's size, shape or exterior appearance, your body is made up of powerfully vibrating energy, and this energy determines what you look like externally. For example, if you look old, fatigued or stressed you will inevitably have a low, possibly toxic energy field vibrating within and around your body, whereas if you externally appear to be vibrant and happy you will inevitably have a glowing energy field that is within and surrounding your body. Whilst you may not be able to see this energy with your naked eyes, it is scientifically visible with a thermal field instrument.

The energy vibrating within your body not only determines how you look, but most importantly it determines how you act and feel, the fulfillment of your potential, your ability to fulfill your purpose, and thus, the quality of your life.

You may not be able to see this energy, yet you can certainly feel it. Upon introspection, you can easily discover when you are full or empty of energy depending on the way you feel. At a simple level, the days when you feel great are the days that you have a high level of virbational energy flowing through you, whilst you have low, slowly vibrating energy when you don't feel so great.

Discovering the Energy Within You

If you close your eyes and sit still you can feel the energy that I'm talking about vibrating and pulsating throughout your body. Try this for a few moments; wherever you are, pump your fists really hard and throw your arms around as if you're really excited. Don't hold back, pretend you've just found the greatest secret to your life's success and that you are so excited that you're throwing your fists triumphantly in the air. Now stop, sit still, close your eyes and feel the energy flowing through your body. If you close your eyes and pay close attention to your left hand, you will be able to feel the energy that runs through you. If you have a deep sense of awareness you will eventually feel that same energy flowing all throughout your body. You will be able to feel energy flowing through every body part as well as the energy of your heart pumping blood throughout your body. Notice the intense vibration throughout your body. Eventually you will be able to feel this energy just by sitting still. The energy that you can feel is not just within you, it surrounds you in a field similar to a bubble. The more vibrant and energised that you are, the bigger this bubble will radiate. The energy that you feel flowing intensely throughout your body is the same energy that flows through every single object in this world – this is the energy of *Universal Intelligence*. The same energy that is in you is *everywhere*. Take a look around you again. The energy that runs through everything that you can see with your eyes also flows through you. There is more to what you can merely physically sense in every life form – everything around you is energy and we are all connected to this same energy. The moment you become aware of Universal Energy is the moment your life changes forever.

More deeply, you are not simply the body or face that you see when you look in the mirror; you are divine eternal, pure essence – you are the energy that flows through you – the energy that connects you to your Higher Power. The energy that flows through you is responsible for the way you show up in your life. You will discover that being mindful of this energy is more important than you could have ever imagined.

The energy that flows through all life forms is more powerful than anything in this world. In fact, *it is* the energy of the world – it is the energy of Universal Intelligence, the Creator and sustaining Power of this magnificent world. The energy of which I speak is so powerful that those who effectively harness it become able to do the seemingly impossible. This energy is responsible for the bond between a mother and her child, it is responsible for allowing karate masters to break bricks with their hands, doctors to heal incurable diseases, athletes to produce extraordinary results, inventors to bring such profound greatness in the world and people such as Mahatma Ghandi, Martin Luther King, Jesus Christ, and Buddha to create such tremendous change in the world. The same energy is responsible for the force of the ocean, the wind and the perfect alignment of the planets, which along with *every* object you can sense, is the Universal Intelligence's expression of energy. Nature *is* Universal Energy and by connecting to nature, you can effectively connect to Universal Energy, thus connect to your higher purpose. When you are connected to the energy of the world, the same energy that created our galaxy, our earth and the human body, you are unlimited in your potential to fulfill your deepest desires.

We each have different levels of energy and are each in control and responsible for our energy levels. You may notice that some people always seem to be happy and energetic. These people have high levels of energy flowing through them, whereas people who always seem to be down, lethargic or even depressed have a naturally low connection to energy.

Have you ever spoken to a friend or relative who was in a bad mood and then all of a sudden felt really drained and down? Or have you ever spoken to someone who was in a really good mood and then all of a sudden felt really energetic, excited and happy? If you take notice from now on you will find that the energy of every single person that you come in to contact with always affects you. Even if you speak to someone on the phone, their energy still has the power of affecting the way that you feel. I will discuss this in detail later.

The implications of energy run far deeper than anyone may have ever thought. 99.9% of all people's actions are determined by their connection to Universal Energy.

When we have high levels of natural energy flowing through us we feel excited, enthusiastic, loving, loved and encompass many positive emotions. With higher energy levels we have a heightened sense of beauty and a feeling of purpose in our lives. With a high connection to energy the body is more efficient, helping us to feel better and be more productive. Conversely, when low on energy we feel negative emotions such as stress, worry, anxiety, fear, irritation, and anger amongst others. Low energy is the number one cause of all illness and disease. If you're currently feeling positive emotions then you are full of positive energy. If you're feeling negative emotions you have low energy levels.

A strong connection to energy creates bliss, whereas a low connection to energy creates all negativity. Everything is created from the same energy, the energy of Universal Intelligence, yet the level and intensity of the vibration of energy determines the quality of an organism's life. You see, humans are like a rechargeable battery. We take in energy and we give out energy. When we are connected to Power we work at full power and full potential. When we are disconnected from Power we struggle to live a meaningful life.

Being unconscious to this fact, people are constantly trying to gain energy in any way possible. Consciously you may not realise that your connection to energy determines how you feel, yet unconsciously everything that you ever do is tailored toward bringing more energy into your life. In every moment of our lives we are either gaining or losing energy. You've probably never realised this, but everything that you do in your life, every single action you make, every single word you speak, every single interaction you have with others, every aspect of your life revolves around gaining energy.

The energy of which I speak influences the large majority of almost every person on Earth and being unconscious of this allows your life to be controlled by external sources, primarily your ego. Lack of Universal energy in humans is the cause of any problem that the world has ever had and any problem that you have and will ever have in your own life. You will never fulfill your potential unless you have substantial Universal Energy flowing through you. This generally creates an inner conflict that inevitably causes negative emotions and symptoms in your life, resulting in a need to mask these emotions through negativity and poor habits such as over eating and alcoholism.

The Creator of this world has provided all humans access to the energy that is required to survive, such as heat and light from the sun, oxygen, water and food. This is all we require to survive, yet we all have a much deeper purpose than mere survival, and humans can only prosper and achieve this deeper purpose if they are highly energised. To put it simply, your connection to Universal Energy determines the quality of your life – not your job, not the amount of money you make or your social status, but your connectedness to Energy. The greatest energy that you will ever embrace comes through connecting to the energy of your Creator and giving your highest potential – your purpose – in greatest service to others. It is imperative that you connect to this energy in order to gain the strength needed to take life's challenges head on.

A BROKEN HEART IS REALLY A BROKEN ENERGY FIELD

The importance of energy is highly noticeable when looking at intimate relationships. One of the reasons we seek love so desperately is that it is the only cure for loneliness, which in itself is a need for Energy.

You may have noticed when you begin a new romantic relationship that you feel an intense connection to your partner. You get excited every time you even think about your partner, have a newfound sense of confidence in yourself and can't wait to tell all of your friends about how great you feel. There is more to what you feel than an intimate or sexual attraction; the great feeling that you have occurs because your energy field connects with your partner, filling you with increased energy and vibrancy. During this time, you are no longer energised by your own energy field alone, but rather you share the energy of two people, which makes you feel vibrant and incredibly happy.

This is one of the best feelings that a human can ever have and is so intense and so great that it becomes addictive for a lot of people. Whilst two people in a new relationship experience this connection they feel euphoric love, intense excitement and one of the highest vibrations of energy possible. This energy vibration is so intense that a lot of people unconsciously seek out a partner just so that they can have this energy flow through themselves. The connection of force between the partners energises and makes them feel *alive*, in fact the most alive that they may ever feel their entire lifetime. For those who previously didn't have a connection with Universal Energy, the energy that they get from their partner replaces the previous void of energy that they had in their life. Even for those who previously suffered depression or severe sadness, life is great when they begin a new romantic relationship.

But have you noticed that eventually, usually after a few months, the initial energy field between yourself and your partner begins to fade? As the 'honeymoon' period begins to turn into a comforting relationship, the energies between yourself and your partner slow to a much lower vibration. You still really like your partner, but the initial excitement and energy that you used to share has faded. Whilst you probably don't realise it, the energy fields that were initially bound together to create one energy field are slowly starting to separate back to each individual. Instead of having the energy of two people, each partner reverts back to having his or her own energy again. This unconsciously causes a stir of emotions within each individual in the relationship. After all, they have become addicted to the euphoric feelings associated with the initial energy shared at the beginning of the relationship and as their energy reverts, they don't feel anywhere near as good as they did when their energy was bound together.

What happens then is the major cause of the breakdown of most relationships. The two individuals in the relationship want more energy from the other, but they are no longer receiving it. Thus, each individual *unconsciously* causes conflict with the other in an effort to draw energy, just as they do in every other area of their life. This process is highly unconscious. After all, every person learns from childhood that when you cause conflict by crying or yelling at your parents, they immediately give you energy, whether that be by cuddling you, talking to you or giving you attention. So each partner habitually causes conflict to drain the other partner's energy in an effort to bolster their own. This is what causes many people to have large arguments and emotional fights with one another after the initial few months of the relationship. Unless one of the partners gains energy by connecting to Universal Energy, they will continually cause conflict with their partner to gain more energy for themselves. In return, if the other partner doesn't gain Universal Energy they will retaliate with yet more conflict, starting a highly negative downward spiral of conflict to the point that the relationship can no longer be maintained. This explains why so many people end up hating each other after they break up, even though they were completely infatuated with each other not so long before.

In summary, when two people form together into an intimate relationship their energy joins together, helping them both to feel highly vibrant and 'on top of the world'. This feeling is generally sustained for a few months, in which time both partners become accustomed to the amazing feelings that the new relationship brings. However, once their energy fields separate and the initial spark of energy fades away, both partners start conflict with one another in an effort to feel the energy that they've become addicted to. This is the beginning of the end for most relationships, especially the relationships where people can't stand each other by the time the break up. A broken heart is really a broken energy field.

The thing to think about with this is that most people unconsciously go into relationships to *gain* energy. Some people even chose partners to make them look powerful, impressive, special and admired in an effort to gain energy by impressing others as a way to make themselves feel good. The greatest way to sustain a long-term, fulfilling relationship is to not go into the relationship looking to gain something. Once you begin energizing from natural sources you will not need to rely on another to energize you and will be able to focus on giving yourself fully to your partner without any ulterior motives. Inevitably, all of your relationships will reflect the relationship that you have with yourself. Great relationships are built on the foundation of unconditional love, and this is only possible with a connection to Universal Energy.

LOW ENERGY CREATES CONFLICT

If you are unconscious to the notion that everything is Energy and that the quality of your life is determined by the vibration of Energy that flows through you, your life will forever be controlled by your quest to always gain more. If you are unaware that you will live an incredible life by connecting to Universal Energy, you will always try to steal energy from others however you can.

I say 'steal' energy because people literally take energy from others without others being aware. Stealing energy is not a crime, yet it is destructive. Humans have an overwhelming underlying need to get energy, and most people do whatever it takes to get it, which is the reason most people try to 'be' someone instead of expressing their truest selves. Some people want energy so badly that they will do what they know to be wrong and some people will even break the law in order to get it. In fact, any conflict that has ever happened in the world has been a battle for energy. Any conflict, whether it be between family members, employees, countries, governments or religions is *always* a battle of energy. The sole reason for conflict is caused by the underlying need for people to steal others' energy to bolster their own because they need more energy to make themselves feel better.

For your mind to easily understand energy, imagine two people are standing next to each other. Both people have their own energy fields that surround them. When one person does something to steal the energy from the other person, what happens is that the field of energy surrounding the victim transfers to the person who is stealing the energy. The victim becomes weakened because their energy has transferred to the person who stole it. In that brief moment the person who stole the energy feels powerful, whilst the person who had their energy stolen feels weak, and is likely to experience many negative emotions as a result.

Conflict is a simple battle for energy. Think about the times that you have the most frequent conflict with others. May I suggest that the times that you argue, fight or have any other dramas with work-mates, friends, family or your partner is when you're low on energy and not feeling great about yourself, when you're tired or fatigued, when you're stressed from work or when you've been surrounded by negative people all day. The reason? When you're low on energy, when instead of having a large surrounding energy field you simply have no surrounding energy field, you want to gain energy any way possible and one of the means to do this is to steal others' through conflict. Your brain has been trained throughout your whole life to gain energy by taking it from others. We learned to get our parents energy from the time we began crying as babies and from then on learned how to gain energy to bolster our own. When we were hungry for food, we learnt that we could get what we wanted by crying. When a parent tends to a crying baby the child literally takes energy from the parent to bolster its own. When you argue with someone you position yourself above them to steal their energy and increase your own, and this is the very reason that arguments ever occur. Whoever wins the conflict inevitably steals the energy from the other, be that very briefly.

It is worth noting again that when creating conflict 99.9% of the time people are not aware that they are trying to gain energy from others. It's also very important to note that one actually suffers from taking others energy, for what you do to others you also do to yourself and any energy that you steal from others quickly releases from your body in a very karmic fashion – there is a much Higher Intelligence that determines this.

When someone says 'You're wrong and I'm right' – the fundamental cause of any conflict – the deeper reason for this is that they want to take energy from the other person. Have you ever had a conversation with someone where you *knew* that you were right, and you argued with another person because they thought that you were wrong? If you weren't low on energy you wouldn't have felt a need to argue with the other person, you wouldn't have needed to prove yourself. Yet something deep inside of you made you push the point – you wanted to be right and prove the other person to be wrong. This is not an argument between two energised people, this is an argument between two egos trying to steal energy from one another.

On a larger scale, any war that has ever been and ever will be comes from one country or religion saying to another 'You're wrong and I'm right'. Inevitably, the person who 'wins' the conflict steals energy from the other. Yet all people who ever have conflict have limited energy to begin with, so the person who wins the conflict rarely feels more energised. I certainly can't think of any countries or religions that were more energised for a sustained period after winning a war.

Simply, no conflict would ever occur if the people of the world realised the significance of connecting to Universal Energy, for these people would have no need to take energy from others because they would already be strongly connected to the Energy that is required to live their lives to their fullest potential.

Ego

Ego is the number one reason why society has reached the point where it is now. Ego = Edging God Out, which is quite literal, as the ego is merely the self made illusion that is created when one is disconnected from Universal Energy. We're on a constant drive to find fulfillment through 'things' and in doing so, have become very selfish. It's time that the world woke up and realised that the continual craving for more is a disease of the ego, which is nothing more than a disconnection from Energy. Your ego stops your true self – your eternal essence – from fully expressing itself to the world through self-sabotage. A need for energy is simply what creates and sustains the ego. Nothing is ever good enough for the ego. It constantly wants more and will never be satisfied. To recognise this is a great thing.

Colloquially, the term ego is attached to someone who is arrogant, bigheaded, or conceited. I'm not talking about any of those definitions. When I speak of ego, I refer to the completely false sense of self that each and every person in this world has. I'm talking about the side of you that constantly holds you back and the voice in your head that is never happy. The character that the ego plays is not you; it's a falsely created, mind-made *delusion* that takes over your true being.

Your ego is an energy hungry, self-made illusion that tries to control your life. It does everything it can to steal energy from others. In doing so, it imprisons you to a certain way of living that doesn't allow you to come anywhere near fulfilling your potential.

Your ego creates a false identity for you and makes you believe that you have to fight with others for energy. Your ego creates the world that you live in. Your ego only identifies with form and makes you believe that your outside is more important than your inside. It tries as hard as it can to possess the mind and create the illusion of separateness from others, controlling the way you act and the way you live. It is the part of you that labels things as 'good' or 'bad' and the part of you that makes you believe that you are limited to being the certain person that you are. You live your life based on who your ego makes you believe you are. For example, you act a certain way in your relationships, your job and your social interactions based on who you think you are. Yet as long as you are disconnected from Universal Energy, this person is illusionary, made up by the ego. Who you think you are is simply a delusion that your ego makes you believe. Who you really are is much deeper than the form which your ego can see.

Your ego is an insecure gremlin who wants to prove itself to be better than everyone else so that it can steal energy from others. It tries it's hardest to stop you from realising that you and everyone else in this world is connected, and is therefore the one thing that will stop you from achieving your dreams and your destiny. By taking you away from your connection to Energy, the ego has you believing that you need to 'have more' and 'be more' because you need to compete against others to look superior and steal energy. This delusion always brings suffering. Your ego is the selfish part of you, the you that always says 'I', 'Me' or 'Mine'. Driven by fear, the ego constantly tries to make you look and feel superior to others. It tries to position itself as being superior by 'knowing' more, 'having' more and 'being' more than others. Because it's driven by fear, your ego makes you want to fight with others to steal their energy. It always wants something bigger and better, and whatever it obtains is inevitably never good enough. Your ego was conceived by fear, lack and insecurity and feeds on conflict, unhappiness and negativity. It needs to create a sense of identity by separating itself from and being better than others. Your ego is what causes you to put others down and feel envious and jealous of others, all as a way to protect itself from its deeply imbedded insecurity. The ego attaches itself to the past and holds on to everything 'negative' from your upbringing, your past environments and cultures to establish a sense of aloneness and identity.

The ego craves energy, thus is responsible every time you are disrespectful, angry, rude or argumentative with others. It is responsible for your blame and resentment. It enjoys making itself right and others wrong. Your ego tries to gain energy by making you look better than others, yet it can never get enough energy to satisfy its cravings. When the ego inevitably doesn't gain the required energy, it resists the current situation by becoming resentful, angry or frustrated. The ego thrives, seeks and relies on superiority to gain a sense of self worth. This explains the reason for the importance that society places on materialism and attractiveness. The ego simply cannot comprehend that the individual gains more energy by connecting with Universal Intelligence and by giving itself to others.

The first step in overcoming the ego is to observe and be aware of its existence. You need to realise that your ego has taken control over your true self and will continue to control your thoughts and actions until you overcome it by connecting to Energy.

Realise that when you act out without integrity that you are not being your true self, but rather, your ego is manipulating you to act a certain way. Your ego will only ever cease to prevail when you are connected to your Higher Power. When you are spiritually connected your ego simply has no power over you and you are free to express *your true self*.

Once you become aware of the ego, you are then able to stop the cycle of striving to acquire and be more than others. Your increased spirituality and awareness of the ego will slowly begin to transcend the fear, lack and insecurity that the ego relies on. Attachment to things as a way of gaining energy will drop away. As you begin to love yourself and your purpose in this amazing world the ego loses its power over you. After all, when you fully love yourself you have no insecurities or fears for the ego to feed off. Even more powerful, if you take the wonderful journey of finding your purpose, your spirit will finally be free from the imprisonment of your ego and its associated obsession with form. You will notice that the ego is nonexistent and thus you will always have total control over your thoughts and actions when you are following your purpose and are in full alignment with Universal Energy.

Lacking spirituality, people are likely to identify with 'things', for the ego substitutes these 'things' to fill the void that comes from lacking a meaningful spiritual relationship. At its strongest – which is when it is fully disconnected from Universal Energy – the ego searches for substitutes for meaning, which explains the reason for the colloquial 'rat race' and 'hedonic treadmill'.

Until you transcend the ego and find greater meaning in life, no person, possession, house or anything else will ever give you lasting fulfillment.

The greatest way to find the meaning that you are craving is to create a spiritual faithfulness and follow your purpose. When you are able to get to this point and see the ego for what it is, you will find that you become accepting and grateful for everything in your life, no matter how 'bad' your ego previously made your life situation seem. When you transcend your ego you'll stop taking things personally, you'll stop feeling a need to become attached to 'things', you'll stop competing with others and you won't feel a need to position yourself above everyone else. Instead, you will simply be joyfully at ease with your life.

When you follow your purpose you are free of ego. Instead of doing things because you want to impress others, make money or acquire power or authority, when you follow your purpose you do what you love, what you're great at and what helps others. You will find that when you are following your purpose you are simply not concerned by the judgement of others because you know from the bottom of your heart that what you are doing is what you were put on this earth to do. There can be no greater motivation or happiness than that which comes from freeing yourself of others judgment and living your life *expressing your true self.*

Transcending the ego

Quite simply, if you want to transcend the ego, become successful, happy, fulfilled and find meaning in your life, you must be willing to connect spiritually and find your purpose. The ego loses all of its power over you once you connect with others on a deeper level because you are no longer identified with the illusionary 'I' that the ego creates. Instead you are functioning from a much deeper consciousness; the consciousness which connects you with Universal Energy.

You may recall that before I was talking about those who are sceptical about the contents of the book. If you find yourself being sceptical about the contents of this book and particularly about what I've just written, it is highly likely that your ego is what is holding you back from this truth. You're ego fears that it will lose its control over you if you begin to neglect what it has previously told you and follow your true destiny. If your ego is holding you back, being aware of its presence is the first step towards transcending it entirely. When you are conscious of the ego, it no longer holds power over you. As long as you are aware of the ego and the illusionary self which it tries to make you believe that you are, it cannot take you over and pretend to be you. Don't lose yourself nor restrict yourself to the ego's mind made illusion. Realise that the ego is not truth and as you do, the essence of who you *truly are* will shine through. Life really isn't as serious as your ego makes you believe it is; feed your ego with positive energy and it will quickly run away.

PRACTICE
- Notice the influence of the ego anytime that you find yourself trying to find fulfillment by being bigger and better than others or feeling resentful, angry or frustrated. Next time you find yourself in conflict with others, question the deep reason for your need to prove yourself to be right and others to be wrong. To overcome the ego, firstly accept that it is there. The more awareness that you bring to the ego, the less power it will hold over you.

DISCOVERING WHAT REALLY CREATES WELLBEING

Before we go any further, I want to challenge your values to help you determine the influence that your ego currently has over you. I want to challenge your idea about what makes you happy.

Does the life that you're currently living hold any significance? Think about this question honestly. Are you living a life of significance?

Does your life have any meaning? Or are you on a constant quest to have more money, more power, more security or more status?

If you were to die tomorrow, would you be happy with your life's contribution?

If you're controlled by ego and not consciously living to your highest potential you'll end up feeling dissatisfied and bound to the traps of society – you'll get sucked into the trap of acquiring more. More money, more status, more beauty, more power and more fame. More, more, more.

The point that I'm making is that, as a whole, society's values have become increasingly geared towards making money and having more possessions as a means to finding happiness and fulfillment rather than towards living a life of purpose. This is the influence of the ego trying as hard as it can to gain *energy*. I'm imploring you to discover that a life of consistent happiness, love and meaning lies beyond the constant struggle to have and be 'more'.

I want you to question yourself; what do you think makes you happy? Do you think that having more money, possessions and status makes you happy? I mean, really?

It's a typical cliché question and deep down I think we all know the answer; if you rely on making money and acquiring 'things' as a way of making yourself happy, you'll simply never be happy. In fact, you will create suffering in your life because you will constantly be using your precious time to chase energy that is unattainable through this method. We live in a world where everyone seems to be on a constant chase for more money, more possessions and more status. The fear of not 'having enough' or 'being enough' seems to have intensified to the point where it has overtaken people's true values and almost turned some people into money hungry robots. Society has reached the point where it now fiercely over values money, looks, security and status and has a barren unawareness of the purpose and quest that each of us has had our lives blessed with. Little does society know that the constant striving to be and have 'more' stems from a lack of connection to energy.

Most people vastly over value the ability of more money and more possessions to bring them more emotional wellbeing. This isn't just my opinion; it's a scientifically proven fact.[3] Despite this, people still think that money and possessions will make them happy. Unfortunately, you're on a nonstop journey to an unfulfilling existence if you search for happiness through anything in form. Deep meaning, happiness and love can only stem from true love for oneself and a connection to Universal Energy.

Sonia Lyubomirsky, the author of the best-selling book 'The How of Happiness' has scientifically proven many times that whilst acquiring money and possessions might lift our spirits for a very short period of time, it does not provide lasting happiness, satisfaction or fulfillment. To chase money, possessions and 'things' is to shrink our soul by not fulfilling our greatest potential.

Let me introduce you to the hedonic treadmill – the constant strive for more.

The Hedonic Treadmill is a theory developed by Michael Eysenck, stating that humans are predisposed by genetics to plateau at a certain level of happiness, and that the occurrence of novel happy events merely elevates this level temporarily.

It is clear that rather than becoming happier as people become better off and acquire more, people's expectations and desires also become greater and rise in tandem, resulting in no permanent gain in happiness. You can compare this method of pursuing happiness to a person on a treadmill, who works harder and harder as the treadmill spins faster and faster, only for the person to stay in the same place. Human beings always want more because of our ability to adapt. As soon as we acquire something, our initial satisfaction steadily declines and leads us to want something bigger and better. Nothing material ever consistently fulfills us because the energy void that we have simply cannot be filled through acquiring 'things' into our lives.

---

3 Nickerson, C., Schwarz, N., Diener, E., and Kahnerman, D.

You may think to yourself, 'If I had X amount of money I'd be happy'. But it has been scientifically proven that once you acquire that extra money, you will be happy for a couple of weeks, only to then lose your initial satisfaction and then want even more. If you earn or gain more money, you will inevitably spend more and then you will want even more again. If you get a pay rise, you'll be happy for a short period, but inevitably you will adapt to that pay rise, your initial satisfaction will dwindle, and you will want an even bigger pay rise. No matter how much money you bring into your life, your energy level will always remain the same over the long term.

Thinking back to your own life for a moment, can you see how no matter how much money that you've earned throughout your life, your expenses have always risen in line with your income? Can you notice how you've always wanted to have or be more, no matter what you've had?

Despite it being completely false, people think that acquiring more money, possessions and status will make them happier and provide them with the energy that they unconsciously seek. If you earn $40,000 you might think that earning $70,000 per year would make you happy. Inevitably, when you do get to that stage that you earn $70,000, your initial satisfaction will be replaced with dissatisfaction which you think will only be cured by earning $100,000. And hence, you blindly jump on the treadmill and work towards acquiring $100,000.

You may one day buy your dream house, but the scientifically proven fact is that two-six months later it is inevitable that you'll want something newer, bigger and better. The rule also applies for cosmetic surgery. Most females who get breast enhancements gain initial satisfaction and renewed confidence from their larger chest, only to feel unsatisfied and crave having even bigger breasts a few months later. You've probably seen photos of celebrities who have had so much facial surgery that they look like aliens, with skin stretched so tightly that they can hardly make normal facial expressions. This is a prime example of adapting to initial satisfaction and wanting *more* to satisfy the ego.

If you ever go to a gym you'll find that no matter how great someone's body looks, they will always want to look better. You may look through a magazine and be envious of an incredible body, thinking to yourself, 'I wish I had a body like that'. But even that person would want to have a better body. The fact is, regardless of how much one has, humans always seem to want more.

If you don't know where you're going and you're simply driven to always have more, will your quest to have more ever end? Will you ever slow down to enjoy the fruits of your labour? Studies show that you won't smell the proverbial roses and will remain on the hedonic treadmill until your working life is over, depriving yourself of freedom and the greatest human trait - fulfilling your potential.

If you always want more and have unlimited needs that are underwritten by a desire to gain a connection to Energy, it is guaranteed that you will never reach high levels of happiness and meaning in your life. Always wanting 'just that bit more' – no matter how much you have – causes constant feelings of limited fulfillment.

No matter what happens *externally* in our lives, human beings always return to a stable level of happiness, which Sonia Lyubomirsky calls the 'Happiness Set Point'. Just like a thermostat always returns to the same temperature even after fluctuating up or down, the same can be seen for our happiness and energy levels. A person who wins the lottery will return to the same level of happiness one year on as if that same person had become a paraplegic. It has been scientifically proven that it doesn't matter how happy or how sad one becomes after a life changing situation, one will always return to same happiness set point – *unless that happiness comes from within.*

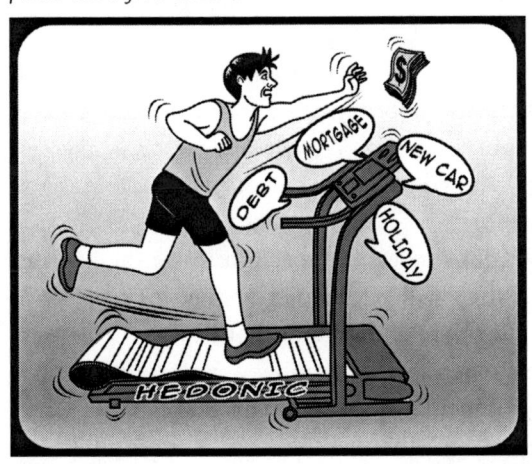

This means that it doesn't matter how much money, possessions, status or power you acquire, your happiness will always return to the same level and your desires and expectations will constantly continue to rise and fall, leaving you with no change in happiness and an invariable desire for *more* – unless you can gain the energy that you seek through connecting to Universal Energy. We can literally compare the pursuit of happiness through acquiring money and 'things' to a person running on a treadmill, constantly exerting energy but not getting anywhere, the carrot always dangling just out of their reach. This is because we always adapt to what we acquire without a substantial change in our connection to Energy.

As a collective society, over the past 100 years we have acquired enormous amounts of wealth, technologies and accessories – yet collectively we have steadily become *less* happy. In fact, in the past fifty years, the GDP of the USA has tripled, yet depression rates have multiplied at least ten fold. Our world has become enhanced in so many ways, yet levels of depression are reaching epic proportions. The contagion of individualism in our world is a massive contributor to the incredibly high levels of depression. This makes sense when you consider that striving to have and be more is a highly selfish pursuit that disallows a connection of energy with others. The reason for depression: your soul wants more. One's soul knows that its capabilities and potentialities are far greater than its current output, and it creates a feeling of depression in an effort to *wake you up*.

One hundred years ago, many of the world's richest people didn't have running water and they definitely didn't have TVs, DVD players, iPods, cell phones, computers, internet or cars. Yet scientific data has shown that as the years have proceeded and as we have acquired more technologies and accessories to 'enhance' our lives, we have literally become less and less happy.

Even if you earn the average income in a developed country, you now have more luxuries than the richest people in the world had fifty years ago. Frank Lloyd Wright once said, *"Many wealthy people are little more than janitors of their possessions."* Are you a janitor to your possessions as you strive to acquire more and more?

People who have aspirations to gain higher esteem through material gain truly believe that they will be happier if they look better in the eyes of others, yet studies have shown that that those who express materialistic aspirations live much less satisfied lives, and are even more likely to develop a variety of mental disorders! This makes sense when you consider that at a deeper level, the one thing that people are trying to acquire is Energy, and that can never be found through any pursuit to 'have' or 'be' more, causing great unhappiness to those who use up great amounts of energy in their pursuit.

Sonia Lyubomirsky also notes a study of over 700 wealthy people which found that more than half of the people who were interviewed reported that wealth did not bring them more happiness. A third of those who had assets greater than $10 million even said that money caused them more problems than it solved. *Ten million dollars!!!* – that would make you happy, right?! Well maybe you'll be happy for a little while, but as silly as it sounds, inevitably you will adapt and want *more*. Ten million dollars simply will not satisfy the connection to Energy that you require to prosper.

Not only does the quest to gain happiness through the acquisition of more money and material possessions constantly lead to unhappiness, it also takes your time and energy away from higher values and joys such as nurturing relationships, fulfilling your purpose, spending time with family doing activities that actually enhance your connection and happiness and enjoying the many gifts that life has to offer.

Exterior wealth is meaningless if you are not rich within. There's no point being a winner at your job if you're a loser at life. Even if you have one billion dollars in the bank, fulfillment will only ever come through the application of your greatest self to a cause greater than yourself. It simply does not matter how much money you have, you will always live a shallow existence until you create a connection with Universal Energy by giving your absolute greatest self and providing meaning to others.

It would be so sad to get to the end of your life and realise that you had opportunities to create a significant difference in this world and offer more joy and love to yourself and those around you, yet you spent your life constantly trying to have and be more – only to fulfill your own selfish desires.

If you feel as if you're stuck in the 'rat race' or on a 'hedonic treadmill', know that becoming aware of this is the first step towards overcoming it. Begin to question your values, question what is important to you, and be willing to search within to find an abundance of love, happiness and satisfaction. Create a connection to Universal Energy. There's a big difference between looking rich and feeling wealthy, and most of the people who look rich aren't wealthy. Those who feel wealthy are those who are connected to the whole. Find something to live for. Follow Leo

Buscaglia's wisdom; "It's not enough to have lived. We should be determined to live for something. May I suggest that it be creating joy for others, sharing what we have for the betterment of humankind, bringing hope to the lost and love to the lonely."

Don't get me wrong; I love money just as much as everyone else. Money is a great energy that flows into our lives when we create value to others. But you are deluded if you constantly try to acquire more and more because you think that it will make you happy. The money and material possessions that you are trying to bring into your life are a cover for the energy that you *need*. Your anticipation of acquiring more objects and possessions is fear-based work of the ego. The energy, fulfillment and meaning that you are searching for will come to you not from making more money or having more things, but through connecting to the Energy of the world and fulfilling your purpose.

If you want more love, more happiness, more satisfaction, more joy and more fulfillment, you will find it when you search within, connect to your purpose and give your greatest energy to fulfill the needs of the world. Barack Obama says, *"Focusing your life solely on making a buck shows a certain poverty of ambition. It asks too little of yourself. Because it's only when you hitch your wagon to something larger than yourself that you realize your true potential."* This book is focused on helping you to realize your true potential and fulfilling the contribution that you were born to make.

PRACTICE
- Write a list of the things that you do to look good, and then write a separate list of the things that you do to make you feel good. Do less of what makes you *look* good and more of what makes you *feel* good.

EFFECTS OF LOW ENERGY
So what happens when you disregard the call of your soul to fulfill your purpose? Below is a list of all of the things that disconnect you from Energy and often fill you with toxic energy. By disconnecting you from Energy, these things all create food for the ego to thrive on.

It is very important to note that we should never judge anyone on the things that they do to gain energy. Everyone wants to live a life of significance. Everyone wants to be special, important and unique and people do the things they do to gain energy and feel good about themselves. Everyone wants to feel significant, and in doing so, everyone has their own way of getting that energy because we all know at a sub conscious level that the times we feel significant are the times that we are full of energy.

Through individualism, violence, tattoos, making money, having possessions or fancy cars or simply playing a certain role, every single action that a person who is unaware of Universal Energy makes is tailored to gain energy. This is why people are selfish – they get greedy and want as much energy as they can possibly have. Understanding why people play these roles allows you to realise the reason people act in a certain manner. Each of the things that I'm about to discuss literally disconnect you from Universal Energy.

Energy Drainers
The obvious things that drain you of energy and often fill you with toxic energy are:
- not getting enough sleep and rest for your body,
- not exercising,
- having a poor diet,
- overeating,
- over consuming anything such as alcohol, cigarettes, refined foods or debt.

These are the common things that drain you of energy at the conscious level. Unconsciously, Energy runs much deeper.

Fear and worry take your energy
Have you noticed that when you are fearful and worrying, your enthusiasm, excitement, love and all other energising emotions become erod-

ed? Fear fills your body with toxic energy, disconnecting you from your Higher Power, for to be fearful is to disconnect from the trust and faith of your eternal essence. Being fearful is a clear sign that your ego is controlling you and that you must reconnect to Energy. Similar to fear, negative thoughts drain your energy and disconnect you from Universal Energy. Negative people suffer unhappy lives. They often repel people. I don't not know any negative people who are happy, vibrant or fulfilled. In fact, scientist Martin Seligman says that being pessimistic is about as bad for your health as smoking two packets of cigarettes a day. Being negative not only drains others' energy, it drains your own. It is impossible to be connected to Universal Energy and be negative at the same time.

Chasing extrinsic goals takes your energy

People unconsciously think that money, possessions, status and power is the energy that will fulfill them. This is what the ego believes and strives for. Once acquired, you find that these things only provide you with a very short boost of energy, only to leave you wanting more. The more that one strives for 'things' as a means of energising, the further disconnected they become from expressing their authentic, eternal self.

Being around energy suckers takes your energy

Have you ever noticed how drained you feel after spending time with certain people, doing certain work or undertaking a certain activity? These things drain you of all energy and often leave you with toxic energy. Some people are so energy deficient themselves that they take all of yours to fill their own void. They do this by complaining, criticizing, blaming others, making you feel sorry for them, boasting, bragging, being selfish and much more. These people diminish your energy field to bolster their own.

 We also have automatic, autopilot reactions when people take our energy when we're not present. Think about any time that someone has been rude to you and stolen your energy. It is most likely when this happens that you will automatically react without even thinking. This is how the ego protects itself. But by doing this, you also automatically create toxicity in your body. As you know, being controlled by your ego disconnects you from your field of potentiality. Motivational speaker Jim Rohn says that you are the average of the five people that you spend most of your time with. Whilst it's hard to avoid certain people, you should always try to spend time with people who energise you rather than suck you dry of all vital energy.

Similarly, whenever you complain, blame, grieve, argue, react to others, are angry, rude, or disrespectful, not only do you suck energy from others, you also fill your own body with toxic energy. Has doing any of these behaviours ever made you feel great? I highly doubt it — it may give the ego a momentary sense of superiority, but that is then replaced with toxic energy. Making yourself feel like you are right and the situation/other person wrong will always drain you of vital energy.

Stressful situations take your energy

Stressful situations disconnect you from Universal Energy. You simply will never be stressed if you are present and accepting of your situation, thus to be stressed is to be controlled by your ego. Stress, which is determined by your relationship with the present moment, creates toxic energy in the body and stops you from being able to function efficiently.

Doing jobs/work that you don't like takes your energy

This is one of the most common energy suckers in our modern world. Doing anything because you 'have' to will always drain your energy. If you don't like your work it is likely that you will complain, blame and criticize others and have negative emotions such as stress, anxiety, fear and anger creating toxic energy in your body every single day. Instead of focusing on doing your work, you'll constantly day dream and drift away from the task at hand, creating constant inefficiency. This is certainly no way to live. You will *always lose energy* as long as you are not presently focused on the specific task at hand.

Watching too much television drains you of energy

As you sit on the couch and watch the screen your mind often gets filled with toxicity of fictitious dramas. Watching too much news is also a massive energy drainer. The media doesn't sell stories; it sells toxic energy that the egos in people love to thrive on. Have you ever noticed how drained you feel after you watch the news? News and other media stories suck you dry of energy, and egos become addicted to it. The ego loves the drama, the hatred, the anger and anything else that is can use to keep you under its control. Also, studies have shown that we breathe shallowly and inconsistently when we watch television. This explains why many people feel grumpy or lethargic after they've been watching television – their bodies have been deprived of highly energetic oxygen.

Menstruation drains females' energy

For females, the time when you're most likely to find conflict is when you're menstruating. The period of menstruation often completely drains females of energy, which is why you get so emotional and often try to steal energy by causing conflict with others. Some women even get cravings – they are so low on energy that their cravings make them eat foods that they usually wouldn't because the body needs energy in any way possible. Females can easily overcome low moods and energy by reenergising through natural sources (explained later) during menstruation.

Here is a list of examples of how being disconnected from Universal Energy can affect people's lives:

People break the law to gain energy

People are capable of doing the most inhumane things to gain energy. Anyone who has ever done anything harmful or stupid had an underlying need to gain energy. Think about any person who has ever done something fundamentally stupid. Anyone who has ever committed acts of crime, deceit and adultery despite knowing that what they were doing was fundamentally wrong, was void of energy and attempting to gain more. The reason for rape, murder and terrorism all stem from the same cause; people who commit these acts of crime are so devoid of energy that they commit crimes that they know they should not just so that they can take energy from their victims. You may think that some people commit acts of crime because they seek revenge. Deeper than revenge lies the underlying need to satisfy the ego and regain the energy that was stolen from that person in the first place. Someone stole their energy and they want it back – that is the underlying issue behind all revenge.

Those who commit crimes or fraud based on an underlying greed and want for power are also void of energy. It is not uncommon to hear of a wealthy man who has been sentenced to jail for committing a crime related to robbery, colluding or inside trading. These people don't commit crimes to gain more money, although that may seem to be the case, they commit crimes because they are void of Universal Energy. Greed is a desire for more, no matter how much one already has, which is only caused by not being spiritually and purposefully connected.

When people steal material goods from others, when arson, rape, murder, or any other crime is committed, the criminal is always void of Universal Energy and committing the crime is their instinctive means to satisfy the ego by stealing energy from others. When a person commits a crime, they not only hurt others, they also steal their energy and gain a sense of significance. No person who is fully connected to the energy of their Higher Power ever feels a need to commit a crime because of their awareness of the Energy that connects all things.

Nearly all cases of people committing crimes strongly relates back to the energy they received as children. The children who always make trouble or get into trouble at school are the kids who generally don't come from loving families. Think back to when you were at school and you will probably remember a class clown or a mischievous child who always used to get into trouble. It is highly likely that this child was not given enough energy at home, whether their parents were abusive, interrogative, intimidating, simply didn't provide enough attention or presence or if the child learnt from an early age that the best way to get energy/attention from his parents was to be naughty. The children who are naughty at school make trouble to gain some energy and significance because it's the easiest way they know how. What generally happens is the child learns that being naughty is the easiest way to gain energy from others, even if the energy is not necessarily positive. This creates a destructive cycle of poor behaviour where the child continually behaves poorly because this is the only way they know how to get energy from others. It is a sad reality that these children generally grow up to be the adults who end up in jail. When they got into trouble at school, teachers and/or parents punished them for their actions rather than realising that the underlying reason for their actions was to gain some sort of significance. Their lives would be completely different if they had been given love and positive energy from an early age.

Obesity is the outcome of low energy

We don't have to look too far to realise that large a percentage of the world is obese. People overeat in an effort to fill the void of energy in their lives. I can definitely tell you that the times when I overeat and indulge in junk food are the times when I'm disconnected from Energy and thus act without integrity and either feel down, tired, angry, irritated or bored. These are the times that I'm low on energy and without knowing it (well I know now) I stuff my face full of food to fill the void. Take notice next time you binge and you will likely find that you are low on energy. Yet the energy that we are lacking and crave can never be found in food. When we are in these moods, it doesn't matter if we eat all day long, we still won't feel fulfilled. People who are overweight or obese crave good energy yet they generally eat junk foods which only fill the body with depleted energy, creating a cycle of even bigger cravings for energy. The excess fat that obese people have on their body is a build up of stagnant, toxic energy. The only way to fill the void that overweight people seek is to connect to Universal Energy.

Adultery and cheating is the outcome of low energy

Narcissism and arrogance are often thought to be the reasons for celebrities, politicians, businessmen and sports stars cheating on their partners. Underlying such causes is the need for energy and satisfaction of ego. This is the same for those adulterers who are not in the public spotlight. These people are so disconnected and have such a great need for Energy that in the moment their need for Energy overcomes the knowledge that what they're going to do is wrong and they risk their entire lives and reputations just for sexual satisfaction. Without ego, people would not act so mindlessly.

People try to make themselves look good to gain energy

People who incessantly work-out or spend large amounts of time trying to make themselves look good *crave* energy. Some people feel a need to be admired and recognised and believe that they will gain the energy that they are searching for through looking attractive. This explains the ridiculously high rates of plastic surgery as well as debt caused from people spending money that they don't have to buy things to be fashionable and impress others. Similarly, people who show off or want to be the centre of attention, people who brag, focus on status and people who want to be famous all crave energy. Our society is quickly becoming materialistic and focused on external appearance. Universal Energy is the only means to change.

Addictions are the outcome of low energy
Smokers, drug addicts and alcoholics all try to cover their energy deficiency through these masking agents. These substances give them a short-term boost of energy that allows them to free themselves of the burden of their mind. Yet all of these substances literally drain vital energy and create toxic energy within the body. In fact, all addictions take over peoples' lives to fill their energy void. Men become addicted to porn, yet not because of the porn itself. They become addicted to the rush of sexual energy that fills a void in their life. Some men even fight when they've been drinking because drinking takes their vital energy and replaces it with toxic energy. They want to fight others not to hurt others but to take their energy.

It is impossible to be 'selective' when trying to mask your emotions and energy levels. By numbing our emotions we actually numb everything, for example, by using masking agents to free yourself from the burden of your mind, you also mask and disallow yourself from receiving positive emotions that come from Energy such as joy, gratitude and beauty.

Anti-social behaviour is the outcome of low energy
Anyone who is ever arrogant, self-centred, conceited or disrespectful towards you is low on energy. Similarly, those who exploit their authority over or bully others and those who blame and manipulate others do so because they are low on energy. If you ever find yourself being the victim of another person's anger, rudeness, bullying or disrespect, understand that they act in these ways in an effort to steal energy from you because it's the only way they know how to replenish their voided energy. The kids who were bullies at school and even adults in the workplace are the ones who didn't get enough energy from their parents when they were younger, and now use this behaviour as a method to steal energy from others. People who display these character traits, bullies in particular, prey on the weak. Just like animals that prey on the weak, there is an intelligence in all of us that can sense other people's energy.

People who lie, especially compulsive liars, have very low energy. Compulsive liars spend their lives trying to impress others by boosting their ego in an effort to gain energy.

People who have suffered pain in the past and been unable to see the greater meaning behind their suffering carry toxic energy with them throughout their lives that affects the way they act. Often people who feel pain live their lives in a certain manner to take energy from others to make up for their own deficit. If you carry pain from the past, it's highly likely that you will unconsciously make others unhappy in order to steal their energy. Perhaps you can notice that you blame others for the things you're unhappy about when you are low on Universal Energy and high on toxic energy?

Understanding human behaviour

It must be emphasised that people don't act in these ways to consciously hurt or make others feel bad. There is no such thing as a 'good person' or a 'bad person'. People make good or bad actions and deeds, but these do not necessarily make them good or bad people. Everyone simply *is*; people only act in certain ways to gain energy and significance in the eyes of others. Every single person is divine beauty. Only our energy levels determine our actions, and as such, we should never judge someone based on an interconnected web of events that have manipulated one's energy level throughout their life. The weak, and by weak I only mean deprived of energy, try to take energy from people. The weak are those who are insecure and perceive themselves to be inadequate in the eyes of others, and nearly all of their actions are an effort to gain energy. The people who cause the most conflict and negative disruptions, from a global scale down to the individual, are those who have been deprived of presence – undivided, focused attention – from those around them throughout their lifetime. Rather than judge, blame or criticize such a person's actions, we must see the wholeness and interconnectedness in one another. We are all divine beauty and are all either an energy giver or an energy sucker at any one moment. We are all the same, only varying in vibration of energy.

We must love each person as if they are our own brother or sister or father or mother. Stop allowing the collective egoic illusion from making you believe that we are all separate from one another. We are all connected in our efforts to gain a sense of significance. Treat everyone with loving kindness as if they were your own blood and flesh, because they are.

Roles that people assume

Most people play certain roles throughout their lives to gain energy from others. The most common roles that people play are that of the Intimidator, the Arrogant individual, the Interrogator, the Distant or Aloof individual and the Self Pitying individual. All of these roles are mind-made delusions of the ego. If you notice that you play any of these roles, contemplate a possible deeper meaning behind the way you show up in your life. Here's a brief definition of each:

- **Intimidators** gain energy from others by making others feel small. By putting fear into others, the intimidator easily steals energy from many people who are low on energy, especially those who are insecure. Just like animals who prey on the weak, intimidators can sense when others are vulnerable and low on energy and thus prey on them. Intimidators are so low on their own personal energy that they will often make others feel really bad in order to gain energy.

- **Arrogant** individuals are low on energy and thus low on self esteem. By creating a 'superior' facade they steal energy from others by striving to make others feel inferior.

- **Interrogators** control people by finding things that are 'wrong' with the way people live their lives. The underlying tone of the interrogator is 'I'm right – you're wrong'. The interrogator loves to create conflict to steal another's energy.

- **Distant** individuals are generally aloof and cold. They create stand-offs by appearing rude and their aloofness creates a disconnection between them and others. These people are rarely empathetic because to be empathetic is to give energy to others, and they are unable to give something that they don't have.

- **Self Pitying** individuals are so low on energy that they try to gain energy from others by having them feel sorry for them. They play the victim and make themselves seem hard done by. When others feel sorry for them, they sense a short burst of energy that has been stolen from the other person.

- **Parents** can either be energy givers or suckers at any one time. Whilst almost all parents have great intentions in their role, many parents actually take energy from their children. Nobody is to blame for this because it's likely that their parents did the same to them. Most parents aren't present when they are with their kids because their energy is controlled by their ego, which has them always thinking about their own lives. How can they be present to their children if they can't be present in their own lives? Instead of giving their children 100% attention and energy (which children *need*), most parents actually steal energy from their children.

Many parents control all aspects of their children's lives because this is the easiest way for them to gain energy and a personal sense of satisfaction. As you become aware of the roles that parents play, you will notice that the more controlling a parent is, the lower their own level of energy is. Children especially lose energy when they see their parents arguing. These dramas are caused from people not getting enough attention as children, which goes back to the way their parents treated them. In fact, the role that anyone plays generally originates from their upbringing.

If your parent intimidated you as a child, it's highly likely that you now play the self-pity role. If your parent interrogated you as a child it's highly likely that you are distant whenever people speak to you. People low on energy struggle to care, give and love because this requires them to give energy, and you can't give energy if you don't have any in the first place. If you feel like your parents didn't give you the energy that you required, perhaps this can help you to understand why.

Toxic Energy

Consistent low energy creates toxic energy within the body, which affects people's lives more than anything else. Period. When the body/mind/soul is low on Energy it needs to steal energy from others to feel significant. This means that lack of Energy controls all thoughts and actions. Here is an explanation of how Toxic energy affects you.

Consistent low energy causes sickness and disease among many other ailments. Every moment your body is constantly regenerating, old cells are dying and in their place new cells are being created. In fact, it is estimated that in seven years time your body will most likely be made of completely new cells (energy) compared to what it is made of today. In seven years your body will be *completely* new. As the old cells die, new cells are created from the energy flowing through your body. Your body renews itself based on the energy it receives. So if the body has negative energy flowing throughout it, it has no option other than to use this energy to regenerate. If the body is constantly low on energy, it will create a dull, aging, overweight, wrinkled, fatigued body. If your body is constantly full of positive energy the new cells with be recreated with healthy, vibrant, youthful energy. So to create and renew a healthy, vibrant body, mind and spirit you *must* give your body high quality energy.

Stagnant energy is another cause of disease. People who have diseases, especially the big ones like cancer and heart disease, have bodies that have been regenerated with poor energy. Cancer cells are low voltage cells – cells are meant to be highly flowing energy, and cancer is caused when the cells are low on energy for a prolonged time. Whether from poor diet, poor thoughts or lack of exercise, the energy in cancer cells has not been renewed and allowed to flow freely. The bodies of people with these dis-eases have been filled with toxic energy that has become stagnant through lack of exercise and lack of regeneration through natural sources. Energy is not meant to be stagnant. Stagnant energy creates problems. Never hold onto or hoard energy, always let it flow. Thoughts are energy that certainly shouldn't be held onto. Constantly hoarding thoughts about the past prevents you from receiving new energy. Energy that you hold onto gets stuck in every cell of your body, creating tension and dis-ease. Holding onto old energy stops you from receiving new energy.

You have energy to give to the world, and when you don't fully express your truest self your energy becomes stagnant like a damned up flood. The damn is burst by the creation of illnesses that have the specific purpose of allowing you to realise that you need to rejuvenate and fully express your energy. Herein lies the problem of the modern health system; doctors are good at medicating symptoms of illnesses, yet often neglect the true cause of the initial illness – the energy that created it. If doctors treated people's energy levels, rather than masking their illnesses with medications, the illness would naturally disappear as the body regenerates newly energised cells.

This is why exercising and healthy eating and fully expressing one's self are so important – they allow the body to constantly renew itself with fresh, highly vibrating energy. Everything in this world is impermanent, including your life and the world itself. Think about it; nothing is meant to live forever; everything has a birth and a death. With this in mind, let all energy flow. Don't hoard.

Toxic energy creates a great environment for the ego. The ego thrives on creating negative thoughts and negative emotions such as irritation, anger, hatred, impatience, nervousness, sadness, and anxiety. Feeling anxious, worried, stressed or fearful, is a clear sign that toxic energy is stagnant within you and that you don't have good connection to Universal Energy. Lack of energy is what disconnects us from the whole, leaving us sad and creating a void which leaves us feeling unfulfilled and always wanting more.

As discussed previously, *everything happens for a reason*. If you ever feel 'negative' emotions due to a disconnection from Universal Energy, view these emotions as an incredible alarm clock that is waking you up and helping you to realize that you need to strengthen your connection with your Higher Power and connect to Universal Energy. Your body gives you these emotions as a great gift to help you to realize that the way you are living is not in alignment with your Highest Energy. Simply, you are out of integrity. These feelings are purposely trying to help you to change what you're currently doing so that you can feel the positive emotions from connecting to Universal Energy.

Lack of energy is the number one cause of depression. People who suffer with depression are so low on Universal Energy that they often cannot find a way out. At the two ends of the scale, high Universal Energy creates vibrant bliss whilst low/toxic energy creates depression. If you suffer from depression or often feel lonely, sad or down, you are disconnected from your Higher Power. I have no doubt that your connection to Energy is responsible for the way you feel, regardless of what has brought you to feel these feelings. The great thing about this is that to release ourselves from feeling low, we simply need to reconnect with Universal Energy.

Being low on energy also creates greed. When you don't have enough energy you will almost always over consume in every area of your life, in particular eating, shopping and making money. This explains why there is growing cases of obesity and debt all over the world. Until you fill yourself with Universal Energy, your ego will control your life through overconsumption.

You may have noticed that it's easy to get out of bed in the morning when you have something that you are really looking forward to. Conversely, think about how hard it can be to get out of bed when you are *not* excited about what you have to do that day. Fatigue and lethargy only affect those who are not on purpose. Energy is quickly drained from you when you do things because you *have* to, not because you *want* to. Aligning yourself with your purpose fills you with tremendous energy, whereas you are much more likely to feel fatigued and lethargic when you are not flowing with Universal Energy.

When you are low on energy people all around you will suffer because you will try to steal their energy, generally by causing conflict. This creates inauthentic and unfulfilling relationships.

Just like everything in life, there is meaning and reasons behind such conflicts and the role playing that produces them. To overcome this, it is so important that you know who you truly are, become aware of the roles that you play and remain present as often as possible. By finding the meaning behind them, you will not only transcend these dramas, you will also overcome the ego.

These are just some of the examples of why the human world is a vast competition for energy and power. It is now time to wake up from the collective delusion of the ego. When you are constantly energised from natural sources, *you do not feel a need* to cause conflict or compete with others because you already have enough energy flowing through you – conflict is simply unnecessary if one overcomes the ego by connecting to Universal Energy. Embracing all that Universal Energy has created, including the deep beauty of oceans, mountains, gardens, loving others and performing many other energy enhancing activities that I will soon talk about, *connect you* to Energy. We can end all human conflict by gaining energy from our Higher Source. This piece of knowledge is literally life-changing.

You can also easily overcome being affected by people who try to steal your energy. Awareness is the first step. Now that you are aware of the importance that energy has on the way people act, you will consciously and deliberately be able to sense other peoples energy. Reacting to others when they act in a particular energy stealing way only ever causes conflict and what generally happens is energy goes to and fro between yourself and the other person as both of you try to gain energy from one another. They take your energy, and then you take their energy, creating a vicious cycle. Reacting instinctively when others try to steal your energy will only continue this emotional cycle. Whereas if you react only with presence, awareness and love to others you will end this cycle and create a new consciousness in yourself and others. The best part of all is that *presence, awareness* and *alertness* created through non-reaction and non-resistance connects your energy field with those who previously tried to steal from you. Instead of energy going to and fro and both people leaving the conflict filled with toxic energy, if you simply respond with presence, their need for energy will instantly dissolve. Your presence connects you to, and evokes, energy in others. And the more connections of energy you share, the more meaningful your life will feel.

Next time someone is rude or mean or does something that makes you want to react, see *if you can pause and create some space between what is actually happening and your thoughts about what is happening.* Look at the facts rather than instinctively reacting. Ask yourself if you are creating a story in your head, or if the way that you perceive the situation is actually real. Become present and see the situation for what it truly is: a simple battle for energy.

The situation will not affect you; in fact, it will energise you if you respond with presence and awareness. Conversely, if you allow the situation to affect you and drain you of energy, you will have fallen below consciousness and back into egoic, instinctive behaviour. Know that every single person comes into our life to either send us a message or teach us something. We must remember this every time we meet someone. Appreciate each and every person because they are in your life for a reason. Give everyone great energy.

With your newfound awareness and consciousness of the reason certain people act the way they do, your will no longer be the victim of other's actions and will no longer allow your emotions to be determined by the way others treat you. You now know that people live their lives in a manner that makes them feel strongest and most significant. The awareness that you bring to your own and other people's needs for energy will certainly allow you to transcend any problems. Power imbalances, selfishness, greed, and other 'negative' traits that others possess will have no power over you and will not be able to affect you with this new awareness. Your life will be incredible when you are able to understand the meaning behind all people's actions and respond to all people only with loving kindness and presence.

Is the alarm clock waking you up yet? If you're feeling empty or lacking the amazing energy that comes from enthusiasm, it's time to make a change and connect to Universal Energy and begin living a life of purpose.

PRACTICE

- Be aware of the things that drain your energy. Perhaps you can notice that you blame others for the things you're unhappy about when you are low on Universal Energy and high on toxic energy?

- If you are overweight, have an addiction, constantly complain, blame, grieve, argue, react to others, are angry, rude, stressed, fearful or disrespectful – notice where all of these are coming from. Be aware that you can end these dramas by connecting to Universal Energy.

- Constantly remind yourself that any negative feelings and emotions that you experience are very purposeful. Your body gives you these emotions as a great gift, a way of telling you that you must change what you are currently doing. Always listen to what your body is trying to tell you.

Fulfilling Your Potential

All living organisms require an external source of energy to survive. After gaining energy from natural sources, organisms then use this energy to live. For humans, at the most basic level the necessary energy required to live includes sun, water, oxygen and food. These are the external sources of energy that humans need to merely survive. But life goes far beyond survival for human beings living in the 21st century. We want happiness, meaning, fulfillment, wealth, health, purpose, spirituality and much more. To live with these conditions we need so much more energy than is available from things like food and oxygen; we need to connect with the amazing energy of Universal Intelligence – the natural energy that abundantly surrounds us and is available to *everyone*.

In order to fulfill your potential and live your purpose, you *must* connect to Universal Energy, you need to stay plugged in to the amazing energy that provides you with infinite potentialities. The greatest people to have ever walked this earth, past and present were all made great because of their strong connection to Universal Energy.

Your level of energy and the level of success that you have in your life is an expression of your connection to Universal Energy. Accordingly, if you want to live a life beyond mediocrity and fulfill your potential you must become aware and allow Universal Energy to flow through you. When you are connected spiritually and live in harmony with that connection, you will then be connected to the Energy of everything that has ever been created. You will feel a vibration of energy that connects you to every single person in this world. When you are connected to the One Power that created everything that has ever been in existence in this world you are connected to every source past and present. You realise that you are not alone and that all the divine beauty that surrounds you is also *a part of you* – a part of your eternal soul that lives on before and after the birth and death of your human body. When you connect with that powerful energy you will hold within yourself unlimited sources of anything that you ever want or need to fulfill your purpose. You will always be assisted by the same Force that grows your fingernails and keeps the sun rising every day.

If you can live your life in accordance with Universal Energy, you will have no limits to anything in this world – nothing will be out of your reach, especially your deepest desires. You will be able to tap into unlimited sources of love, happiness, creativity, talents, wisdom and much, much more. You will come to the point where you can acquire everything that you need to fulfill your purpose, even if what you need comes from unknown sources. If you need creativity but aren't a creative person, you can be sure that someone highly creative will come into your life to help you. If you don't have enough money to fulfill your purpose you can be sure that someone will come into your life to help you raise funds. If you need specialised knowledge or help, you can be sure that you will draw from unlimited sources to find that help. If you feel like you do not possess enough intelligence, imagination, talent or any other intangible asset that you need to be 'successful', know that if you need these assets in order to fulfill your purpose, *you will acquire them* by becoming one with the tremendous power of Universal Energy. One can even become a genius by connecting to this energy. The power that comes from connecting with the same energy that created and maintains this world *cannot be overstated.*

Fulfilling your potential by listening to and acting on the deep drive that lies dormant within you is by far the greatest way to connect to Universal Energy. Have you ever wondered how some of the greatest businesspeople to have lived have built such magnificent companies without attending or completing schooling? People like Henry Ford, Thomas Edison, Albert Einstein, and Andrew Carnegie all never finished High School. Yet they seem to have unlimited creativity and genius. There is simply no way that these influential people could have achieved these amazing successes by themselves. They all went that one inch and then even further beyond mediocrity with help from what they received from their connection with Energy. Whether they knew it or not, these great people connected to the Oneness of all life forms by listening to and then expressing the sound that raged inside of them. They all had faith that they were destined to win, to achieve and to express the nature of their Source. Mahatma Ghandi is another amazing person who achieved amazing things in his lifetime from being fully aligned with Energy. He said, "I offer you peace. I offer you love. I offer you friendship. I see your beauty. I hear your need. I feel your feelings. My wisdom flows from the Highest Source. I salute that Source in you. Let us work together for unity and love." Ghandi knew that he was spiritually connected to every person to have ever lived, and drawing from unlimited sources from within that Energy he was able to *change the world*.

Faith

In writing his best-selling book titled *Think and Grow Rich*, Napoleon Hill spent twenty five years studying over five hundred of the world's most successful people and found that faith was one of the most important characteristics that successful people hold. Hill says, "*Faith is the head chemist of the mind. When faith is blended with the vibration of thought, the subconscious mind instantly picks up the vibration, translates it into its spiritual equivalent, and transmits it to Infinite Intelligence (Universal Energy), as in the case of a prayer.*" Hill says that faith is the "'*external elixir' which gives life, power and action to the impulse of thought*", "*the starting point of all accumulation or riches*" and is "*the only agency through which the cosmic force of Infinite Intelligence can be harnessed and used by man.*" Napoleon Hill dedicated his life to creating a formula for success and found that one's union with a Higher Power is vastly important.

If it sounds unrealistic to you that great people of this world are only great because of their connection to Universal Energy, know that I was once similarly sceptical. Once again, a spiritual world cannot be physically or scientifically proven, but I assure you that any highly successful, spiritual person will agree with what I'm telling you. The unlimited resources available to those who maintain a strong relationship with Universal Energy are nothing short of remarkable. I would not have had the ability to write this book without the unlimited resources that I'm telling you about. I've got no training in writing. What I do have though, is a strong spiritual connection and an amazing energy flowing through me which is generated from following my passions and my purpose. Everything that I needed to write this book always came to me, including people who brought me inspiration, ideas, funds to continue writing and much more. Inspiration 'just comes into our head' often without searching for it. Anything great that has ever been created in this world has come from a flash of inspiration or intuitive insight, and this inspiration comes from a connection to Universal Energy. I implore you to tap into these unlimited resources and find out for yourself – there's an abundance available to every single person in this world.

Any person who has ever accomplished something great in his or her life has done so through the expression of their deepest inner drive, which connected them to the unlimited resources provided by Universal Energy.

To that end, we should stop relying on our conscious mind to make our big life decisions, such as what we should study at university, which career path we should follow or which job we should take. Our brain can weigh up pros and cons only with limited and manipulated social knowledge. Much more powerful than the brain alone, the subconscious mind that is connected to the power of the Energy of this world will *always* guide you in the right direction and allow you to make decisions based on what best aligns you to your purpose. When you do tap into these resources, you will find that you are always in the right place at the right time and whatever you need will always come to you. You will also find that certain people, circumstances and events will come into your life at the perfect time to help you, reminding you that we are connected to an Energy much greater than the mind can comprehend. It is almost as though everywhere you go you know that you are being helped and guided when you have this connection. Everything that you do seems to be easier than previously. Quite simply, every moment during your day becomes a vehicle for consciousness. The assimilation of this knowledge is incredibly powerful.

Not only does your connection with Universal Energy determine how successful, meaningful and effortless your life will be, it also determines the emotions that you feel every single day.

Whenever you feel passionate, excited, enthusiastic, happy, loved or any other positive emotion, it comes from a connection to Universal Energy. These feelings are a sure sign that the way that you are living your life is in accordance with your highest integrity – what you know to be true. The times that you feel extreme bliss, fulfillment and satisfaction are the times when you are completely aligned with your highest potentialities. As you free yourself of ego (the greatest resistance against living an incredible life) your life will become an effortless glide towards fulfilling your purpose. You will feel creative, energetic, healthy, alive and highly vibrant. You will gain an enhanced perception of beauty and discover that your perception of beauty in all forms is an indicator to your connection to Energy. As you become strongly connected even your senses will become enhanced and you will find greater beauty in all that you can see, taste, touch, smell and see. Starry nights will fill you with joy, water dripping off plants after it's rained will fill you with a sense of connection to the whole and viewing blue skies, green grass, trees, plants and other natural beauty will become incredible spiritual experiences.

Those who don't fully love and express theirselves need to steal energy from others to fill the void that is missing in their life. By connecting to Energy you will learn to fully love and embrace yourself and in doing so, give tremendous energy to enhance your life as well as the lives of many others.

Your life will truly become incredible when you are fully aligned with Universal Energy. When you've fully aligned yourself with Energy you will be living the life that you are meant to live – not the life that you think others want you to live – the life that Universal Intelligence created you to live. Aligning with this path, this energy and power is by far the greatest thing that one can ever do with their time on Earth.

Finding Your Purpose

By far the greatest way to connect to Universal Energy is to fulfill your deepest inner drive; your purpose. This is your one obligation in life. Your purpose is what you have been put on this earth to do – the reason why you were born into this world. It is what the Creator of humankind has always planned for you from the very moment that you came from nothingness into this world of form. Obey this obligation and you will be granted with a meaningful life.

The person who you are and the events that have shaped your life in the past have always been leading you towards your purpose. Each and every person on this planet is here for a reason, just as every event in your life happens for a reason. The world is very purposeful. You must know that there is a reason behind absolutely everything, and there is a reason for your life. There are no accidents. There is a Universal Power that flows through all of us and is helping us all to fulfill our purpose. Your purpose isn't necessarily 'big' – not everyone is going to have the same large scale impact as Martin Luther King or Mahatma Ghandi. Your purpose may be to be an incredible parent, teacher or nurse, or to bring joy to people through the arts. Your purpose is highly important regardless of the size or scale of reach – every single person has an important role to play.

Don't be mistaken by thinking that finding your purpose is a Holy-Grail chase. Your purpose is dynamic – changing as your life evolves.

Your purpose is spiritually charged and you will find that once you find your purpose you will have an Energy running through you unlike anything you have ever felt before. If you want to feel that power and live the extraordinary life that I've been talking about, your job right now is to find your purpose.

In the following chapter you will find questions that specifically allow you to find your purpose. Answering the questions to find your purpose is a process of interviewing your soul. The questions are designed to allow you to realise *your true self*, a knowledge which is greater in value than anything money can ever buy. The questions will help you to discover and realise your truest values – the values that have been lying under the smoke screen of values that society has ingrained in you. The questions will help you to realise what is most important to you; making money or connecting with others; work or wellbeing; a life of possessions or a life of meaning.

By continually answering these questions, you will eventually receive answers from your subconscious mind – the part of your mind that knows who you truly are beyond what your friends, family and society want you to be. It is widely thought that your subconscious mind is directly linked to Universal Energy. By continually questioning your subconscious mind you will receive answers from the energy of your Higher Power – the Power that created you – the Energy that gave you your purpose and has always been leading you toward it throughout your entire life.

I cannot stress how important answering these questions is. You need to look deep into your heart to truly awaken to the power that you hold within. You weren't born into this world to idly wish or dream – you were born to awaken you true greatness and shine it upon those who are lucky enough to be blessed with your gifts.

Putting in the Required Energy

Johann Wolfgang von Goethe famously said, *"Things which matter most must never be at the mercy of things which matter least."* It is now time for you to start putting tremendous energy into the things which matter most in your life. By now you know that fulfilling your purpose is the most important thing you can ever accomplish in your life.

Finding your purpose requires regular work and practice. To use a metaphor, trying to find your purpose is in many ways similar to being fifty pounds overweight and trying to get back into shape. Just as an overweight person has gained weight from years of poor discipline and bad habits, we are the same with our minds. All throughout our lives we have been conditioned to strive for the things which 'matter least'. Your job is to now condition your mind to connecting with Universal Energy and finding what matters most – your purpose.

If you were fifty pounds overweight you wouldn't expect to go to the gym a few times and get back into shape straight away. The same applies with finding your purpose. I've put together some extensive questions for you to answer in order for you to find your purpose. Please don't expect to answer the questions once and think you'll find your purpose. If you're overweight, you will get back in shape by taking diligent, patient, persistent and playful action. To lose weight you need to push beyond the point of comfort. If you don't push your comfort zone you'll never change. If you want to gain all of the amazing benefits of finding your purpose, you also need to take diligent, patient, persistent and playful action. Why do you need to be playful? It's highly important that you enjoy the process. As with anything in life, the journey and present moment always brings greater fulfillment than the end goal. If you spend your precious time on Earth waiting until you get to a certain point in your life to start enjoying yourself, will you ever really be happy?!

In the long-run, if an overweight person does nothing to change their life in order to become healthy; they will continue to live an unfulfilled existence. They may even suffer health problems. The same is true in your quest to find your purpose. It's your choice whether or not to break old habits and create a highly fulfilling, meaningful life. As long as you don't fulfill your potential, you will always have an inner conflict from being out of integrity.

I used to read lots of informational, motivational self-help books and never really acted on what I read, until one day I realised that it doesn't matter how much knowledge you accumulate through reading, it's all mostly pointless until you dig deep to find your true self. If we want to live a meaningful life, we each must really discover exactly who we each are and what we truly stand for. You can read all you want, but you won't gain anything unless you're willing to do the work to put it into practice. Your growth depends upon your ability to put in the required effort.

Your higher intelligence wants you to show it how important this is to you, thus you need to consistently put in the time and effort to answer these questions. You're not going to find the answers after one journaling session – this is a process. Just like the stone cutter hits the rock hundreds of times before it finally breaks, you too must be willing to put in considerable effort.

Albeit that I didn't have this sort of learning tool when I was in search for my purpose, it took me about two months of constant journaling, questioning and meditating to discover what my true passions and strengths are, what my purpose is, and how I can use my purpose, my passions and strengths to make a living. With this learning tool, it will take you even less time to find your purpose. Realistically, it might take you one month to find and start living your purpose.

There can be no doubt that doing one month of self discovery so that you may live a lifetime of fulfillment is a very good deal. Playfully, persistently, and patiently asking yourself these questions *will* set you up for a life time of happiness and end the suffering that you've previously had. One month of your life will set you up to live a life that feels like a non-stop holiday. One month of your life will allow you to do work that you love every day for the rest of your life. It is well and truly worth it – I know from experience. Interestingly, the answers that you seek will come to you much more quickly when you have a strong connection established with Universal Intelligence.

It is so important that you put the required effort and energy into your quest of finding and living your purpose. Approach life as a classroom and have a growth mindset rather than a 'reaching a destination' mindset. Know that growth comes from work and effort. Change will happen, but we need to change our mindset about it happening overnight. Over time, the benefits of the effort that you put in to finding your purpose will be extraordinary. Are you willing to put in the time and commitment?

Act Now!
At the end of the day, the choice is yours whether to remain in the current circumstances that you are living now, or to do the inner work that will help you truly live a greater life. If you're not happy today then you simply cannot expect to be happy tomorrow unless you begin to make some changes now.

It is a fact that those who achieve only mediocre success throughout their lives are the ones who always wait for the 'time to be right' to do anything meaningful. Lacking courage, these people tend to procrastinate and alas, they never achieve any noteworthy success because the 'right time' never ever comes.

Conversely, people who achieve great success know that the best time to act on anything worthwhile is NOW. It is widely accepted that successful people are the ones who are willing to do the things that unsuccessful people can't be bothered doing. They don't wait for others to come into their lives to make things happen for them – they take a leap of faith, they muster up the courage to get things done and *make things happen by taking action in present moment.*

Self knowledge is the greatest knowledge that you will ever acquire. The questions put forward are designed to help to know yourself deeply and find what is truly important in your life. By questioning your consciousness, you will be able to find not what you *think* you are, but what you *truly* are. If you want to live a truly meaningful life, it is so important that you know who you are. Nobody can tell you who you are, and if you don't know who you are you can't fulfill your greatest potentialities. We all have an unexpressed potential – the exercises are specifically designed to help you find yours.

Unfortunately, many of us aren't aware of our unique gifts. We start our lives with such confidence, love for life and desire to do something great in the world, but as time goes by our uniqueness and our special abilities slowly get smothered by our parents, family, teachers, friends and society who all think they know what's best for us. For you to shine your unique light you must disregard the person you *think* others want you to be and begin to discover your values, passions and strengths and start embodying them every single day.

The questions are divided into different sections, starting with the topic of passion. It must be stressed that nobody can do this for you. Your purpose lies deep within your subconscious and only *you* can tap into that source. In saying that, be playful as you answer these questions. It must also be stressed that the first few times that you ask yourself these questions you will receive answers from your ego. Typically people find it difficult to answer these questions at first. Your ego knows that answering these question will enhance your life to the point that it will be overcome, so it tries to do everything it can to stop you from finding your answers. However, if you continually ask yourself these questions you will go beyond the ego and receive answers from the part of you that has the greatest connection to Universal Intelligence – your subconscious mind. Get yourself a blank journal and be ready to start changing your life.

DISCOVERING YOUR GREATEST PASSIONS

Finding your greatest passions is the first step towards discovering your purpose. Whatever gets you excited or enthusiastic is something that you are meant to be doing – it is aligned with your purpose. As I explained before, when you are enthusiastic or excited, you literally have Universal Energy flowing through you. The things that you are passionate about connect you with that Energy, creating power and liveliness to flow though your body, allowing you to do what you previously thought to be impossible. Following your passion is the quickest way to feel deep contentment.

Think about any person who has ever created something that seemed impossible. Thomas Edison, Mother Theresa, Henry Ford, Martin Luther King Jr. and many more have all manifested the seemingly impossible. How? These people all had an energy field running through them that allowed them to create such greatness in this world, and that required energy was created from strong passion and love for what they did. The happiest and most joyful people in this world are those who have created their lives so that are free to follow their passions regularly. Life grows with happiness and meaning for people who follow their passion every day, especially when they use their passion to connect with others.

If you want to succeed at anything in life then you're going to need to put in lots of effort. To put in the required effort and push through the times that most people would end up quitting, you need to be fuelled by an energy source that can only be found through passion.

Have you ever questioned where passions originate from? Think back to what you really enjoyed as a child. You will find that no one implanted their passions upon you, and how could they? You simply loved doing certain things – that's how you were born, that is what you were made to enjoy. Everybody has unique passions, and the only place they originate from is Universal Energy.

If you are confused about what passion is, passion is simply something that drives a strong feeling or emotion inside of you. Passion is one of the highest vibrating forms of energy. It is energy unlike any other. In fact, passion, love and enthusiasm are some of the greatest energies in this world. Discovering your passions will dramatically increase the significance and meaning in your life.

You will feel a dramatic shift in your being once you have discovered your passions and begin to organize your life around them. You will be filled with energy and will want to use that energy to do your absolute best at everything you embark on. You'll find that it is so easy to do things which you love. Not only will you feel great inside once you start incorporating your passions into your life, you'll also become much better at what you do.

In order to live your greatest life, your aim should be to do absolutely everything to the best of your ability. You simply cannot do something that you don't love to the best of your ability. You want to be putting your whole heart into what you're doing – not being reluctant. With the incredible energy gained from living a life of passion, you will *want* to do everything that is put before you. Rather than living a life of conflict and contradiction where you do things because you feel like you have to, you can craft a life where you only do what you truly want to do. This is the end to procrastination and resistance in what you're doing. In fact, the sense of empowerment as you strive for worthy and meaningful goals will take you further than you could ever have imagined.

Have you ever noticed that when you are doing something that you really love you put much more effort into it? It's terribly hard to do that which you don't like. You may be able to relate to a certain job that you have to do at work.

Can you notice that when you really enjoy a job you put more energy into it, but when have to do a job that you don't like you only put in the minimal effort needed to complete it?

You will come to realise that your purpose is strongly linked to your passions. Universal Energy gave you these passions so that you may use them for the greater good of the world, and at the same time, to fulfill all of your potentialities. Everything is connected.

What if you could create a life where you immerse yourself in your passions all the time – a life where you don't need to do the jobs that you don't want to do? Well, I'm here to tell you that you can and that by finding your passions you will gain the required energy to create that life. Make a stand to not be like most of the people in this world who are willing to spend their days doing things that they don't really like. It's up to you to realise that you no longer need to live that meaningless life. You have the choice to create a life with sustained passions – a life where you have the energy that drives you to do incredible things and create a truly amazing existence.

Highly passionate people are highly energetic whereas those who lack passion generally also lack energy. If you feel like your life is lacking passion and energy, you're not alone. In fact, I'd say that 99% of the world is neglecting full use of this great gift. Nobody can be blamed for this. After all, they never seemed to teach us about following our passions in school. If you feel like passion is absent from your life, see if you can find the seeds of opportunity behind such absence. If you're lacking passion, your body is trying to tell you that you need to make a change. Maybe you need to change your job, relationship, or environment. Whatever the case may be, you need to make a change and allow the strong fuel of passion to flow through your life.

Not only will embodying a life of passion help you to find your purpose and achieve in whatever you do, it will also provide you with incredible health benefits. Living your passions results in creating a positive energy for your body and mind. You'll feel happier much more consistently when you do what you love. Stress – the number one cause of all illness and disease will decrease, leaving you less likely to become sick and much more likely to consistently feel vibrant and energised. With this positive vibration flowing through your body and mind you'll be inclined to exercise more, you'll eat more healthily because you'll feel good about yourself, decreased stress will lower your blood pressure; even the quality of your sleep will improve. Then because you're exercising more, eating more healthily and getting better quality sleep, you'll feel happier and want to continue following your passions. It's a tremendous cycle.

Now that you know that discovering your passions is absolutely paramount to discovering your purpose and creating an amazing life, these questions will help you to realize what you're most passionate about. Write each question individually in your journal or on a blank piece of paper and then write whatever comes to mind. Journaling these questions will allow you to slow your thoughts, increase your focus and tap into the subconscious mind. Your conscious mind is a filter to the subconscious mind, and by writing your thoughts on a piece of paper you are able to slow your mind to the point where it is possible to get through the filter and gain direct access to the part of your mind which runs direct energy between your soul and Universal Energy.

What do I absolutely love in life?
List anything that you *love* about the world and the people in your life. This can be absolutely anything; music, sport, cooking, teaching others, learning, watching movies...*anything*. Within your love for these things lies deep passion.

What gets my juices flowing?
Think about any activities that get you excited and enthusiastic and make you feel most alive. List every single thing that makes you feel happy and radiantly energetic. This list can include absolutely anything. Don't hold back, just write!

What am I naturally curious about?
Think about the topics that interest or fascinate you, the things that you like to read about, the people that interest you, the TV shows and movies that you like to watch. Whatever you naturally gravitate towards is something that you are passionate about.

What is something that I think is wrong about the world that I would like to change?
Think about the things that really annoy you in this world. This question will help you to discover what you truly care about. If you get angry about something, it shows that you are emotionally charged and thus passionate about the topic. So once you discover what in the world annoys you, you can turn it around and provide a service to change whatever it is that you don't like.

As stated earlier, it could take you many attempts to find your passions. Your ego will try to stop you from receiving *your* answers. The answers may not come to you straight away, so be willing to ask yourself these questions every day until you receive answers from your subconscious mind. Once you've found your answers you will know for sure what you passions are. Trust your intuition. This is a large step towards finding your purpose and living an extraordinary life. Now, on a separate piece of paper, write 'My passions are...' and write down all of your answers. Now that you are aware your passions, you can start to implement them into your life more frequently.

DISCOVERING YOUR GREATEST STRENGTHS

As part of your time on Earth and the purpose that you were born to give the world, you have been blessed with some great strengths. Every single person has been given unique individual strengths. What I'm saying is you are really good at something, so great in fact that you could be the best in the world at that thing.

Before we go any further, I can already imagine thoughts running through your mind such as, 'I'm not good at anything' and 'What a joke – as if I'm the best in the world at something'. But the fact is you are!

If you want to find your purpose and live an incredible life, you must release this type of thought about yourself. It's time that the world stopped letting society determine how we all think and feel. The collective ego of society makes us want to feel small, to not boast accomplishments or shine our strengths upon the world, and when we do, society is quick to bring us back down to their level by labelling us arrogant, conceited or big headed.

Step outside your comfort zone, release the judgement you think you will receive from others and be willing to acknowledge your strengths. To realise that you have been blessed with amazing strengths to give to the world is a great step towards finding and living your purpose.

Embracing Your Greatness

You have greatness lying dormant inside you that is yearning for you to express it to the world. It is time to start fulfilling your potential. From the 2nd century Roman Philosophers such as Seneca to modern day leaders such as Martin Seligman and Deepak Chopra, many of the great thinkers and philosophers acknowledge the fact that we each have unique strengths and that the use of these strengths constitutes towards living a meaningful life.

We are born to fulfill our deepest drive, and our lives become *extraordinary* when we do. If you don't bring forth what is inside you – that is to say if you don't use your strengths and fulfill your purpose – your spirit slowly becomes destroyed. It's yearning for you to find yourself, so bring forth what's inside you and save your soul and your world by unleashing your potential. If you don't, your strengths will counter intuitively eat away at you and create inner illness. What you can be, you must be – you must bring forward your strengths and fulfill your potential if you want to live a meaningful life. Become everything that you are capable of becoming, find delight in doing the things that you were made for and give your gifts to the world by utilizing your incredible strengths. Most importantly, be willing to *fully express your truest self*, for your truest self is Universal Energy's ultimate, most beautiful creation.

Using Your Strengths

Have you ever found that when you do something that you're really good at – no matter what it is that you're doing – you find it so easy that you'll happily do it even if what you're doing is something as lacklustre as cleaning, doing chores or an odd job at work?

There is no doubt that you produce your absolute best results when you do things that you're good at. You are bound to be successful if you do what you're good at every single day for the rest of your life.

Forget about improving your weaknesses, focus on using and improving your strengths. We've been given strengths for a greater purpose and must utilize them in order to fulfill that purpose. If you use your time and energy to correct your weaknesses, you may bring them up to an average or mediocre level, yet if you use similar time and energy to further enhance what you're already great at, you can improve that skill to a level where you may be one of the best in the world at that skill. Don't get me wrong, we all have weaknesses that may need improvement from time to time which as humans we need to address. But don't spend too much time trying to improve your weaknesses – they don't serve you. What you were created for and what serves you are your strengths, so direct your focus to those whilst making sure that your weaknesses don't hold you back.

Whatever you do that is beyond your strength level is 'too hard'. Whenever you do things that are too hard, you'll find yourself constantly feeling anxious and stressed. When you can turn that around to doing things that are within your strength level – things that you are really good at – you'll become fully immersed in what you do, living in the moment, in the zone and fully energized. Once you are able to bring yourself to this level of operation, you will find yourself living with high levels of emotional satisfaction and happiness.

Using Your Greatest Strengths in Greatest Service

Once you have found your strengths, the next step is to use them to create a connection with others and provide value to society. Your strengths have been given to you so that you can fulfill your purpose, and your purpose is to provide value to the world – to give of yourself so that the world is a better place because you have lived. Appreciate the skills that you have been blessed with – these strengths allow you to create meaningful and fulfilling services to others, intensifying your connection to Universal Energy.

The simple fact is that you cannot and will not feel fulfilled unless you contribute to and connect with others. It doesn't matter if you acquire millions of dollars, own many properties, travel the world, or have the freedom to do whatever you want with your life, **you will never truly live a meaningful life until you contribute towards the betterment of others** – and I would concur that living a meaningful life is of paramount priority to all human beings.

When I talk about giving yourself to the 'world', I don't necessarily mean that you have to provide a service on an incredibly large scale. You don't have to become an author, politician, public figurehead or anything else remotely like that. Your world might be your family, your community group, your sporting club or your workplace. Everything is connected, so as long as you are giving yourself to someone or something, then you will be creating a service to the world.

There are a number of reasons why giving our strengths to the world helps us to find meaning in life. Firstly, the fact that our body produces 'happy hormones' such as serotonin and we become happier the more we give to others proves that we are born to give, rather than receive. One of the true beauties of life is that you can never help another person without truly helping yourself. Through giving our strengths we also gain a sense of confidence in ourselves, a feeling of connectedness with those whom we help and a feeling that we are making a difference in other people's lives. To give our strengths is to express our true selves and fulfill the significance of our existence.

So gain that sense of connectedness with the world by giving it your greatest strengths. As discussed earlier, you enter this world and leave this world with nothing material and the quality of your life is measured by what you give and contribute to others. It can be difficult to imagine that you are great at something and especially difficult to imagine that you are better than others at something, but your doubts will be erased once you begin to complete the activities below. It's time to deepen your connection to the world and unlock your special gifts!

Questions

By far the greatest way to find your strengths is to take Dr. Martin Seligman's FREE online VIA Character strengths test at Authentic Happiness – http://www.authentichappiness.com. This thorough test will help you to discover your greatest strengths. I, along with over one million others, have taken the VIA Character strengths test and found it highly beneficial.

Go to the website listed above and register your name, then take the 'VIA Survey of Character Strengths'. The test will take 15 minutes and truly help you for the rest of your life. Then, grab your journal or piece of paper and answer the following questions:

What are my best qualities?
List every single thing that is great about yourself as well as all of the things that you're really good at.

What are my greatest accomplishments in life so far?
List all of the moments that you are proud of as well as the times that you've succeeded. To have accomplished these you would have used some of your key strengths. See if you can identify why you succeeded.

What comes to me effortlessly?
List any activities, hobbies or anything else that you do that you complete with ease. Within these lie great strengths.

Similarly to the passion questions, the answers to these questions might not come to you straight away. It's common for someone to ask, 'What am I best at?' and struggle to find an answer instantly. Your ego doesn't want you to think that you're great at something – making you feel little is the best way for it to hold power over you. But as you ask yourself these questions consistently and patiently, you'll find that your subconscious will tell you what your greatest strengths are and how you can use them more in your life. Once you receive your answers, next to where you've written your passions, write 'My greatest strengths are...' and list your top 5 greatest strengths.

DISCOVERING YOUR DEEPEST VALUES

We can't physically see values but we know that they exist. Similarly, we can't see the enormity that lies below the tip of an iceberg, but we know that it exists there beneath the water. Just as the part of the iceberg that you can't see has control of the fate of its tip above water, it is your underlying values that determine the direction that your whole life takes. If you don't take the time to define your values your life will be controlled by your ego and other nasty external forces.

Your personal values have shaped you into the person that you are today. If your goal is wellbeing, you must live in accordance with your highest values, highest integrity and highest potential. **Your life will feel empty of meaning if you don't live in line with your values.**

When we are disconnected from Universal Energy we chase things that are not in integrity with our deepest values. Maybe you work for a company that is unethical, or maybe you work long hours and spend less time with your family. Maybe there are a lot of other things that you do that go against your values. Answering these questions will help you discover who you are and what you stand for so that you can give *your* greatest self to the world.

If my life had absolutely no limits and I could have it all and do whatever I wanted, what would I choose to have and what would I choose to do?

List what your perfect lifestyle would look like. List what you would do throughout the day if you knew that you were bound to be successful, what kind of person you would be, how much money you would make and where you would live. This question allows you to realise who you would truly want to be if there were no limits. By aligning with Universal Energy – the Power that gave you these desires – you can begin working towards the life that you truly want to create. Remember that you wouldn't have a desire if you didn't also have the ability to fulfill it.

What would I stand for if I knew no one would judge me?

List *everything* that you would do if you weren't afraid, even your wildest dreams.

How do I feel when I create for someone else something that I didn't get enough of as a child?

The things that you feel you didn't receive enough of as a child are generally the things that have built a deep drive within you to want to create something in the world. This is often a way of healing a struggle that you may have been holding on to since childhood.

Using myself as a personal example, my purpose comes from seeing my parents unhappy in their jobs. I saw my family members working their butts off and being unable to feel consistent happiness. I constantly heard my family complaining about their jobs. With the knowledge that everything happens for a reason, this led me towards my purpose, which is to help people find their purpose, to find work that they love and to fully express their truest selves. The things that happen to us in our childhood form the people who we become and often determine the direction that our whole life takes.

What do I want to change about specific people in my life?

Is there a certain person or people in your life that you always think about for negative reasons? For example, I have an old friend whom I used to unintentionally think about every day. I thought about how selfish he was, how narcissistic he was, how ego driven he was, how insecure he was and how little he loved himself. At the stage I wasn't aware of the power of Energy. Every single day I would think about this person and want him to change. Then after months and months of thinking about this person, I realised that he was in my life for a reason. He was in my life to clearly point out what I am most passionate about and what I most want to accomplish. It turns out that this friend was part of my life because he was helping to guide me towards my purpose. My purpose involves helping people to find more love and happiness, which indirectly helps people who are disconnected from Universal Energy and who are thus selfish, narcissistic, ego driven and lacking love for themselves.

This is a really big question for you to ponder. Which people in your life (friend, previous friend, family member or acquaintance) do you feel passionately about changing. Is there someone in your life who really annoys you or makes you angry due to the way they behave? Within the thing(s) that you want to change about this person *lies your purpose*.

What would I like to hear people saying about me at my funeral?

Try to imagine that you are at your funeral (playfully). List the things that you would like to hear people say in their speeches about you. List how you would like people to remember you, the legacy that you would like to leave behind, the things that you would like to accomplish, the impact that you would like to have on your family and friends.

This is a big list of questions, so answer them step by step so that you don't become overwhelmed. You should be able to notice some themes as you write the answers to these questions. The themes are your deepest values – the things that are most important to you. The answers that you receive from these particular questions allow you to discover the *true you*, all of your capabilities and most importantly, all of your potentialities. This is highly important stuff! Next to where you've written your passions and strengths, write 'My deepest values are...' and write your top values.

DISCOVERING YOUR DEEPEST DESIRES

These questions are designed to really get your juices flowing and see what really fires you up.

What would I do if I had one billion dollars?

List everything that you would really love to do if you had all the money in the world. Ok, so you would probably travel the world, buy a few holiday houses, do lots of shopping and give some money to your family. Then what would you do? This question helps you to think without limitations. When we are able to remove limitations and boundaries, we can discover what we *really* want to do. Instead of thinking 'Oh, there's no point writing that because it's impossible,' (putting limitations on yourself), write down what you would dare to dream! Whatever you write down is important to you, and is thus important to connect with.

If you had only one wish, what would it be?

Once you have listed your greatest wish, think of a wish that you would like to give to your closest friends and family. If you could give them each individually one wish, what would it be? Is there a trend in the wish that you are giving everyone? If you can find a trend, it is very much aligned with your purpose. Your answers to these questions will further show you what you value, how you would like to live your life and what is truly important to you. This is important. List them with your other qualities.

DISCOVERING YOUR GREATEST INSPIRATIONS AND MOTIVATIONS

Who do I admire most in the world?
List your greatest inspirations and the qualities that you admire about these people. Think about what really inspires you in this world. There is a great reason why you are inspired by certain qualities in certain people. What you admire about others is also a quality that is in you. Whatever attracts you to these people are qualities that you also have. Know that you admire someone because they have similar qualities to you. The qualities that create your connection with these people are within you for a reason, and are a part of your purpose. Whatever you admire about someone else, you also hold within yourself. List your greatest inspirations and motivations with your other qualities.

As stated above, you can't expect to answer these questions once or twice and find your answers straight away. Essentially, you are tapping into your subconscious to receive the answers to these questions. It's going to take time, but it is well and truly worth it.

Receiving your answers to all of the questions is the first step; the next step is to use your answers to find your purpose. This is where journaling becomes highly important. You cannot expect to find your purpose unless you put in the required effort and journal as often as possible. I suggest spending 15 minutes every morning to write out the questions and respond with whatever comes to mind. Don't think about your answers, just write. Be open and non-judgemental.

Continue to ask yourself the questions every day until you've created your list of your top passions, strengths, values, desires, motivations and inspirations. Once you know all of these great characteristics about yourself, you will then be in the fantastic position to find your purpose. Journal the questions presented below every day until you find your purpose. Trust that you will discover your purpose if you continue to practice diligence, patience, persistence and playfulness – and know that there is no better day in your life than the day you discover your purpose. The next step is to bring all of your characteristics together by answering the following spiritual questions.

DISCOVERING YOUR SPIRITUAL ESSENCE

Ask yourself any of these questions as frequently as possible. ? know all of the qualities that make you who you *truly* are. Through this knowledge and by answering these questions, you will find the reason that you were born into this world.

What am I here to do?

What is my mission in life?

What are my greatest dreams?

Why was I born into this world? Why was I born in the year that I was?

How can I create a valuable service?

How can I give myself to the world?

If there was no money in this world, how would I best serve humanity?

How can I find the courage to express my own original ideas?

How can I use my passions, strengths and values to make a living?

WHAT IS MY PURPOSE?

Get emotional. Get enthusiastic. Don't think, just write. If you can't think of anything, just wait – you *will* receive your answers; you just need to be patient. Journal and meditate about these questions as often as you can. When you clear your mind, you create space for you Universal Energy to flow through you. The more you can quieten your mind and allow Energy to flow through you, the quicker you will find your purpose. Ask yourself all of these questions every day with the faith and trust that you will receive the answers when you are ready. You know how important this is for your life, so be willing to keep trying.

How do you know when you have found your purpose?

When you have been given the answer to how you can use you passions, strengths and values to provide service and connect with others, you will have found your purpose. You will know if you have found your purpose because there is no greater feeling. Trust in your intuitive thoughts. Deep down you *will* know that 'this is what I'm meant to do'. When you discover your purpose you'll feel excited, happy, elated and incredibly radiant. It's a feeling so great that you will never forget it. You will suddenly realise that everything that has ever happened in your life has led you to where you are now on a specific quest for this purpose. You will realise the divinity of the world as you discover that the reason for you birth was to fulfill this purpose. You will feel intense energy and excitement every morning that you awaken knowing that you get to spend another day creating greatness for the world. You'll stop worrying about things which matter least and put all of your tremendous energy into using you radiant self to create what you are truly most passionate about. You'll trust in your purpose, you'll trust in the Universal Energy that is running though you and your life will feel magical.

Once you've discovered your purpose, you'll know exactly how you're going to use your passions, strengths and values to create a highly valuable service to the world. You will be willing to produce massive amounts of work without ever feeling fatigued. As you progress with your purpose you will grow more and more brilliant. You'll find yourself wanting to spend as much time and energy as you can fulfilling your purpose and will gain more and more energy with every moment that you are aligned with it. You'll discover little hints and guidance along your journey, confirming the knowledge that your Higher Power is conspiring to assist you throughout every step – this is a feeling that's better than winning the lottery!

Write down your purpose and remind yourself of it every day. This is your life – the life that you are *meant* to live.

KEY POINTS

- You will never live a truly meaningful life until you contribute towards the betterment of others.

- By continually answering the purpose questions you will eventually receive answers from your subconscious – the part of your mind that knows who you truly are.

- Don't leave important things until one day. Those who achieve only mediocre success throughout their lives are the ones who always wait for the 'time to be right' to do anything meaningful.

- When you discover your gifts through specific self contemplation you will find your purpose and mission on earth. Your one and only job right now is to search within yourself to find these.

- Following what you're passionate about connects you to Universal Energy and allows you to bring your highest self to all that you do. Consistently using your passions allows you to live a life where you create a truly amazing existence and have the energy that drives you to do incredible things.

- What you can be, you must be – you must bring forward your strengths and fulfill your greatest potential if you want to live a meaningful life. Be willing to *fully express your truest self*, for your truest self is Universal Energy's ultimate, most beautiful creation.

- Find your purpose and begin living the life that you are *meant* to live.

- If you haven't already answered the questions, do them now – nothing is more important.

Further Connecting to Energy

To further increase your ability to express your deepest inner drive and purpose, the following section allows you to enhance your connection to Universal Energy. I spoke earlier of the incredible feelings one has when beginning a romantic relationship and joining energy fields with a partner. Joining energy fields with Universal Energy in all areas of your life intensely multiplies these amazing feelings by connecting you with the energy field of the whole.

Your connection to Universal Energy must be your primary goal in life. All of your actions must become secondary to fulfilling your reason for existence. To further fulfill your highest potential, you must be in your healthiest state of body, mind and soul. All of the activities that I mention will enhance your energy and wellbeing so that you are able to live at your highest capacity. You will find that as you get to peak energy levels and are vibrating at an exceedingly high rate you will gain thoughts and coincidences from Universal Energy that continue to lead you towards your purpose. You will have more flashes of inspiration and more intuitive feelings.

The activities that I'm about to describe allow you to continually *grow*. If you're not growing, you're dying – it's clichéd but it's true. Think about trees and plants for instance. When they are no longer growing, they're wilting away. The same applies to humans; if we are not on a path towards growth, we on the path towards – you guessed it, death. You have an opportunity to grow closer to your destiny in every moment. Growing energises us in a peculiar way. Ultimate energy comes from fulfilling your potential, your reason for existence, and every single activity allows you to fulfill your potential in every area of your life. Each of the following activities listed will allow divine Energy to flow through you, allowing you to connect with your Higher Power and fulfill your highest potential.

LIVE IN THE PRESENT MOMENT

Being present is one of the most effective means of connecting to Universal Energy. If you're present, you can connect with energy and joy *no matter* what you do. The mind needs to be still and free of thought in order to connect with the energy that *every moment* has to offer us. Within every single moment lies a gift for us to discover, and when we are present we can take what the moment provides us with, but when we aren't present, we miss out on what the world is trying to *give* to us because we are consumed by the ego and its demands. Stilling your mind allows Universal Energy to flow through you, thus allowing every thought and action that you make to be an expression of Energy, whereas if you don't allow Universal Energy to flow through you all of your thoughts and actions will be an expression of your ego. Energy is all around us – being present allows us to connect with it and soak it all in. Most people spend the majority of their time thinking about the past or future and neglect the *now*. Meanwhile, their minds are filled with thoughts and emotions that generally only lower their energy.

Embracing Your Past

Sometimes for those who lack energy at the deepest emotional level, the only way to reenergise and reconnect to a life of happiness, love and fulfillment is to go back into your past, to the very moment that you were born, and discover that everything in your life has always had purpose and meaning behind it. Everything has always happened for a reason. Run through your mind anything that has stopped you from being the person who you want to be. Think of any negative, bad, painful or sad events and situations in your life that have created anger, grief, pain, resentment or guilt. Each of these situations were divinely created to help you grow – even if it takes you many years to yield the lesson that your Higher Power is teaching you. Each of these events offer lessons that provide you with the strength that is required for you to fulfill your unique purpose.

What you must realise is that the past is gone. Incessantly thinking about the past will generally only ferment your anger, guilt, shame or resentment from things that you wish had not happened. Thinking about the past generally cannot provide you with any real benefits. The past is gone. It is now time to realise that whatever happened in the past had meaning behind it and that it has shaped you to be the great person that you are today. Likewise, incessantly thinking about the mind-made illusion of the future will generally only bring your worry, anxiety, stress and fear. Your ego is strengthened when you give more energy and attention to the past and future than the present. Your ego will always try to stop you from being in the present by creating perceived problems in the past and future because it knows that it will lose its power over you if you are present. Constantly being in the present defeats the ego because it simply cannot survive when you are focused on *now*. The only control you have over the future is the level of presence that you bring to this current moment. Connecting with energy will create joy now and in the future, whereas losing energy now will create a disappointing future. You will lose energy in every moment if you are not present. If you are not present you will be a poor parent, friend, employee and partner because you cannot give yourself fully to something if your thoughts and energy are elsewhere.

Everything always has and always will happen for a reason – for a much greater purpose than the human brain will ever be able to process. Release any emotions that are preventing you from expressing your truest authentic self by seeing the greatness and the wholeness of the amazing process of life.

Embracing Your Future

People are so busy worrying about the future that they neglect the present moment. For example, pay close attention next time you eat something that you really enjoy, whether that be chocolate, ice cream, or any other food. See how focused you are on the present moment. If you are like most people, once you've taken your initial bite, you will be thinking about the next bite. You will probably even think about getting a second serve before you've even finished your first bite. The same goes with money. No matter what we have we always want more, to the point that we neglect the goodness that can be found *now*. Even the world's richest billionaires want *more*. We miss the full energy that the chocolate that we are eating *now* brings us through enjoyment and happiness, and instead place our thoughts on the future and miss out on this energy. And this doesn't just stop with chocolate and money. Human beings have become so entranced by what they want in the future that they neglect the wholeness of the present moment whatever they're doing. For example, If you're reading a book, driving your car, eating a meal or doing anything else mundane and your mind wanders off to thinking about what you are going to do at a later time, for example, what you are going to have for dinner that night, in that instant you miss out on the gift that the Universe is providing you in that moment – you miss out on receiving energy and growth that is provided to you in order to help you to fulfill your potential.

The energy that you give to the present moment determines the quality of your future. There is no such thing as an ordinary or mundane moment; every moment holds beauty, joy and energy for those who connect with it. The present moment provides you with the opportunity to build the foundations for a lifetime of fulfilled potential, whereas not being in the present moment restricts your life in many ways.

Conflict

Most of all, not being present prevents you from fulfilling your potential because to do so, you need to be fully energised. And if you don't fulfill your potential you will always feel unfulfilled and lack meaning in your life, with your mind in a constant state of conflict.

Aside from the conflict, you simply cannot enjoy anything anywhere near as much as possible when you're stressed, and the only way you will ever become stressed is if you are not aligned with the present moment. Stress comes from opposing and resisting the present moment rather than accepting and embracing the present moment. For example, we become stressed when another driver cuts us off because we resist that action. We become stressed when we've got a pile of work on our desk because we don't want this to be the case. Stress is caused from opposing rather than embracing such examples.

Of course, it is imperative that you plan your life to create attainable goals and work towards building a life that you want, but in doing so your emphasis must be on what you can do moment to moment. The quality of each of these moments determines the quality of your future.

When you allow your mind to feel anger, guilt, shame, resentment, worry, anxiety, stress or fear, you are absent to the beauty of the now. As discussed previously, you feel these emotions for a reason – your Higher Power is trying to get you to *wake up* and help you to start living in the present moment. Universal Energy provides you with these emotions as a catalyst to change.

Being Connected

Presence allows you to quiet your mind, and in doing so, connect to Universal Energy. When you are present you are free of all thoughts in your mind and your sole focus is on the now. When you are present rather than absently involved with thoughts about the past and future, you begin to open yourself to the beauty of the whole world. Life simply flows with joy and ease. When you realise that every single person, plant, and everything else in this world is the creation of your Universal Energy, you feel a sense of connection with everything that surrounds you. Even the most mundane activities bring you joy. As you walk down the street, you feel happiness and inner peace knowing that the same power that created the grass, the flowers, the rocks, the water, the people...everything – also created you. When you live in the *now* you realise that if Universal Energy is capable of creating such an amazing world, it's surely going to look after you.

If you've ever looked out into green fields, the ocean, a flowing river or a starry sky and felt a sense of awe and amazement, in that moment you were present. In that moment you dropped all judgement, labelling and thinking and connected to Energy. You created stillness in your mind that allowed the great energy of whatever you were looking at to flow through you. In that moment, the Universal Energy and power that was in the form that you were looking at connected with you. You weren't just looking at an object, your energy field was connecting with it.

I vividly remember taking a train ride through one of the most beautiful places in the world, the French Riviera and noticing that nearly every person on the train wasn't even taking notice of the beautiful crystal blue waters and the amazing landscapes that surrounded them. The same thing happened when I was riding a train through the Irish countryside. The endless rolling green fields were breath-taking, yet no one was even taking notice! Simply, their minds were focused on other things (most likely things that they were planning to happen in the future) and were unable to connect to the powerful energy that the present moment had to offer.

There is little wonder why the most expensive and demanded resort rooms are the ones that face the sea, a river or mountains. One would never sit in a bare room and stare at the walls for hours on – imagine the boredom – yet people happily stare at a magnificent view for long periods of time because of the connection of Energy that they feel. When you are on holiday away from a hectic, stressful lifestyle, the space and stillness that is created from looking at these Universally made wonders brings you to the present moment and connects you with incredibly powerful energy. You simply cannot connect with such beauty unless you are present and by being present you are much more capable of accepting and appreciating everyone and everything around you.

Enjoying the Journey

As you become present you begin to release the importance that you previously placed on getting things done. Instead of continually focusing on finishing a goal and reaching a destination, you allow yourself to be lost in the joy of the journey, the present moment, the now. You will do things because you simply enjoy the 'doing' instead of what will come at the end. Instead of being focused on where you are going, your focus shifts to enjoying every moment of the journey. Because you know that you are connected to Universal Energy and that your purpose has already been written, you come to realise that this moment is all you really ever have, and that the only moment to create your greatest life is now – the past is gone and the future is not yet real. The only way that you can fulfill your purpose is to connect with Universal Energy by being present in every moment.

If you're not in the present moment you are never fully here, you are never fully living because you're always trying to get 'somewhere'.

Being present means that nothing is ever a means to an end, which also means that every moment provides meaning for you. Thinking about your life, are there many things that you do simply for enjoyment, or are most of your actions a means to an end? Is your job a means to making money to pay the bills and supplement your lifestyle? Do you eat just to gain energy? Do you exercise just to feel and look healthy? Do you drive your car just to get to a destination? I hope not. The destination that you are trying to reach is always **secondary**. The only thing of importance is *this moment*.

are present you immerse yourself in what you do and in
nothing else matters. You work to enjoy each moment and
is a secondary reward. You exercise to feel the vibrancy of
take and health comes as a secondary reward. You eat to
enjoy the ... and amazing flavours and textures of the food that Universal Energy has provided you with and energy comes as a secondary reward. Rather than each action simply being a means to an end, every single moment of your life becomes extraordinary. Food tastes better, views seem more beautiful, comedy becomes even funnier, and positive emotions intensify.

It is when you release attachment to your mind and your ego that you will fulfill your potential. A mind with constant thoughts and emotions cannot receive energy. When you observe the ego resume your presence, alertness, acceptance and connection. Find your consciousness and spaciousness. Rise above the ego. Allow your life to be ruled by your essence – the part of you that survive beyond birth and death – and magic will happen in your life.

Achieve More

Being present allows you to do extraordinary things that you would never thought you were capable of. When your mind is cleared from clutter and connected to Universal Energy, nothing is impossible. You may often hear athletes talk about how they were 'in the zone' when they achieved outstanding results. 'In the zone' is nothing more than pure presence. The world's greatest thinkers create their best work from a field of pure presence because creativity comes when the mind is quiet, present and energised. I know for certain that the times when I think of the best ideas are the times that I've have escaped the imprisonment of my mind and am fully present in whatever I'm doing.

You will bring yourself to the point where you will find joy and peace, regardless of what you do. There is so much calmness within the present. There are no problems and no stresses in the present.

Presence Exercise

Stop what you are doing for a moment, sit up straight, close your eyes and focus on your breathing. Breathe deeply. Don't think, just focus on inhaling and exhaling for five breaths. Once you have done this, individually place your focus on each of your senses. Focus on what you can hear. Focus on what you can smell. Focus on the darkness at the back of your eyelids. Focus on your body. Sense the calm that flows through your body as soon as your focus shifts from the past or future to the present moment. Your fears for the future and your anger from the past hold absolutely no power over you when you're focused on the now. Noticing your breath – no matter what you're doing – brings you to the present moment. Also, noticing the energy that runs through your body anchors you in the present moment. Feel the energy of your inner body as often as you remember. This allows you to be fully aware of everything so that you may make peace with the present moment. Making peace with the present moment erases *all* problems. Watch your breath, feel the silence and stillness. This creates stillness in you.

When you are present, nothing can steal your energy. It doesn't matter how rude someone is to you, it doesn't matter if you've just crashed your car or if your house has been robbed, none of these will ever affect you if you are fully present because you can see each event has its purpose as part of the connected whole. When you are present there simply are *no problems*. Your present energy also changes the energy of all the people who surround you. If people act in a way that is meant to steal energy from you and you are non-reactive, accepting and appreciative, people will feel much calmer and much more energised around you. As corny as it may sound, this is the way to create a better world.

When you are present, it's not what you do that brings you joy, it's the energy that connects you to Universal Intelligence that allows you to feel joy. To be alive is to be in the *now*. Life becomes amazing when you view the world not through the eyes of the past or the future, but the eyes of now. When you can bring yourself to be constantly living in the now, you simply *will* enjoy every moment of your life. You'll feel a deep spiritual connection with the world and allow the power of the Energy to flow through you. If you are aligned with Universal Energy by being present, life will *always* guide you towards your greatest destiny.

Constantly ask yourself what your relationship with the present moment is. This moment is all you ever have. The past is gone and is now a memory. The future is a mind made illusion which you have only very limited control over. If everything that you do is focused on *this moment* you will discover an extraordinary life. Be present and connect with the energy all around you. Connect with Universal Energy and feel the awe and wonder that this magnificent world has to offer.

Don't Delay Your Life

Before we go any further, I want to make sure that you are living in the now, rather than delaying your life for 'one day'. If your ego has been controlling your life in the past, it's likely that it's taken over your ability to enjoy life *now*. The ego holds fears about not 'having' or 'being' enough in the future. Thus, it forces you to work harder and harder, creating an increasing importance for working towards the future and reducing your ability to enjoy yourself *now*. You cannot be completely happy and content with the present moment as long as you fear what will or won't happen in the future. Your life is void of essence if you don't spend the majority of your life enjoying the present moment. After all, the past is gone and the present doesn't even exist. All you ever have is *now*, and there is no better time to enjoy your life. However, you simply do not realise this when your ego is controlling your life, and inevitably spend your years working towards one thing after another, and then the next thing, and then the next (hedonic treadmill), until one day you die. Your time in this world is limited and the way you use your time determines the quality of your life.

In order to create a meaningful life, focusing your mind to find joy in the present moment is paramount. Do you really think that there is a pot of gold waiting for you that is worth sacrificing the best years of your life for? Are you putting your life off in a constant struggle to be bigger, better and have more? If so, you have two choices: continue to allow your ego's insecurity and fear of lack to overcome you to the point where you keep putting things off until 'one day', continue to live a meaningless life and miss the entire point of human existence, **or**, embrace your life right now and start living your life to your greatest ability and fullest potential.

So many people work tirelessly, doing things that they don't like for the sake of achievement for more than 40 hours per week and miss the best years of their life in the process. And what for – to survive? Not really. In developed countries you can comfortably survive on less than the average income if you release all attachment on unneeded materialistic goods. People often justify their lifestyles by saying, 'I need to make more money to pay the bills.' Yet the bills are high because they have been over consuming in products and services that merely fulfill the ego. The reason why people work such long hours doing jobs that they don't really like, making money to buy things that they don't really need is simply to satisfy the ego. The ego fears that if you earn less money you'll be a 'nobody'. Don't you find it ridiculous that what people think of you often becomes more important than expressing your truest self, following you true mission and living your *greatest* life? Instead of doing what everyone else thinks you should do, follow what makes you feel truly alive. Enjoy the freedom of being who you are by living life on your terms. What is the point of working longer hours to make more money if you are only going to end up having less time to enjoy your life?

Let me share with you an old tale to illustrate my point.

Mexican Fishing Tale
An American tourist was at the pier of a small coastal Mexican village when a small boat with just one fisherman docked.

Inside the small boat were several large yellowfin tuna. The tourist complimented the Mexican on the quality of his fish and asked how long it took to catch them.

The Mexican replied, "Only a little while."

The tourist then asked, "Why didn't you stay out longer and catch more fish?"

The Mexican said, "With this I have more than enough to support my family's needs."

The tourist then asked, "But what do you do with the rest of your time?"

The Mexican fisherman said, "I sleep late, fish a little, play with my children, take siesta with my wife, Maria, stroll into the village each evening where I sip wine and play guitar with my amigos. I have a full and busy life."

The tourist scoffed, "I can help you. You should spend more time fishing; and with the proceeds, buy a bigger boat. With the proceeds from the bigger boat you could buy several boats. Eventually you would have a fleet of fishing boats. Instead of selling your catch to a middleman you would sell directly to the processor, eventually opening your own cannery. You would control the product, processing and distribution. You could leave this small coastal fishing village and move to Mexico City, then Los Angeles and eventually New York where you could run your ever-expanding enterprise."

The Mexican fisherman asked, "But, how long will this all take?"

The tourist replied, "Fifteen to twenty years."

"But what then?" asked the Mexican.

The tourist laughed and said, "That's the best part. When the time is right you would sell your company stock to the public and become very rich, you would make millions."

"Millions?...Then what?"

The American said, "Then you would retire. Move to a small coastal fishing village where you would sleep late, fish a little, play with your kids, take siesta with your wife, stroll to the village in the evenings where you could sip wine and play your guitar with your amigos."

....

The tale puts a lot of things into perspective. If you look closely you will likely find that all that you need to make your life happy is within your reach *right now*.

Ask yourself, 'Why do I work?' Do you work to fulfill your purpose, help others and create greatness in this world? Or are you on a constant selfish quest to be bigger, better, have more and be more? If you are on a quest to have and be more, you will get to your deathbed and realize that you wasted the best years of your life searching for the best years of your life. Don't wait until it's too late to realize that the happiness that you were always striving for has always been *within* and readily available to you.

Another effective method of transcending the ego is the prospect of death. As discussed through the life of Steve Jobs, people are often known to dramatically change their values and attitudes when they face a near death experience. It's as though near death experiences put everything back into perspective. Without making this morbid, I ask you, if you were diagnosed with having a brain tumour, would you still continue to live the way that you are right now? Would making money seem so important to you? Would you care about having and being more? Would you care about impressing others? Or would you care more about expressing your authentic self and making a difference in the lives of others?

Whilst I was travelling throughout the USA I met a man who had just been told that he had a brain tumour and only a short number of years left to live. After initially mourning his upcoming death, he decided to start living his life to its fullest potential. He quit working at his unfulfilling job, he ended his unfulfilling relationship, sold all the unnecessary status ranking possessions that he'd hoarded over the years and decided to travel the world. He made a pact to only do things that he found meaningful. The thought of his imminent death dramatically enhanced the quality of the final years of his life. Would this lifestyle be sustainable if he wasn't going to die soon? Of course it would.

Once you make a shift to becoming a spiritual being you will realise that you come into this world with nothing material and you also leave with nothing material. Don't wait until you're lying on your deathbed to realize that you've spent your entire life searching for meaning by identifying with possessions, when all along the meaning that you've been searching for has been available to you through connecting to the Energy of the world. The completeness and extra meaning that you're looking for in your life is and always will be inside – not outside – you. If you've ever seen an elderly person who is close to death you will discover that because they're about to die they release all attachment to materialism, possessions and money, and are instead filled with love, giving and a sense of spirituality. I implore you to realise this now – not when you're about to die – realize now and stop using your life as a means to an end. **Begin embracing life now**. With life so impermanent and limited by time, I implore you to stop avoiding the things that you really want to do. Live the life that your innermost self wants you to live. Follow the deep drive within you to fully express yourself in every aspect of your life.

PRACTICE

- Begin to do more things simply for enjoyment rather than as a means to an end.

- Whenever you catch yourself drifting into thoughts about the past or future, remind yourself to shift your focus to the present moment. Where possible, integrate the lessons from the past and your awareness of the future into the present moment.

- Use your breathing to anchor you into the present moment. Every time that you notice yourself breathing, quietly praise yourself for being present.

- If you ever feel angry, stressed or any other unfavourable emotion, take a few deep breaths and realise that your actions can come from one of two places; your presence or your ego. The choice is yours.

INTEGRITY

If you want to live a meaningful life with a strong alignment to Universal Energy, the next step is to live in integrity with your highest ideals and values and thus, fulfill your upmost potential. To live in integrity means to do what you know is right in every single moment. On the scale of things that you can do to live a life of constant fulfillment, happiness and optimum energy, living in integrity is extremely important.

For something that is so hugely important in our lives, integrity is a topic that also does not get much air time in our society. If you live your highest integrity you will not only become connected to Universal Energy, you will become healthier (you'll lose weight), more productive, you'll achieve your goals and you will experience far fewer negative emotions. After all, your life's contentment is determined a great deal by the degree to which you express your *truest* self, and living your highest integrity allows you to do this.

To live your highest integrity is to live and act always upholding your highest values and doing what you know to be true. Living your highest integrity means having the self-discipline to forgo the quick fixes and short term gratification for a greater gain.

If you don't live your life in accordance with your highest values, not only will you have constant conflict in your own mind, you'll also live a highly shallow existence.

Nothing is more important than being true to yourself. You know that you cannot 'psyche' yourself into feeling consistent emotions of energy, happiness and fulfillment. The only way to feel consistent happiness and meaning in your life is to act in ways which align with your truest principles and values. Most people live their lives based on the values of others rather than their own values. This causes a constant conflict in one's mind and contributes to the large levels of unhappiness, non fulfillment and depression in our world. To live a life based on another's values is to live a life out of integrity with oneself.

Ask yourself, do you live your life based on what you truly enjoy and stand for, or do you live your life based on what you think will impress and gain others' approval? Are you honest and reliable with yourself and others?

The Integrity Gap

To put it simply, you are living in integrity when your behaviour matches up with *your* values, beliefs, ideals, what *you* say and what *you* know to be true. Coined by Brian Johnson,[4] The Integrity Gap is the gap or difference between what you know to be true – your truest values, beliefs and ideals and the way that you are showing up in your day to day life through your thoughts, actions and deeds.

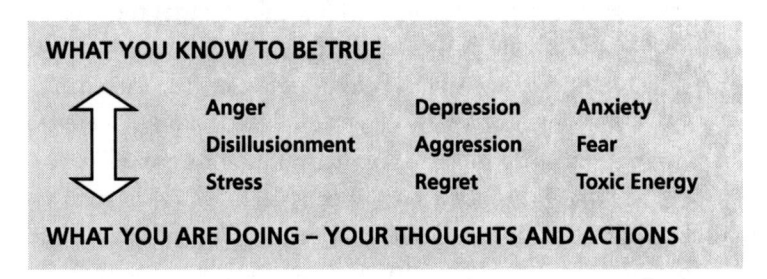

WHAT YOU KNOW TO BE TRUE		
Anger	Depression	Anxiety
Disillusionment	Aggression	Fear
Stress	Regret	Toxic Energy
WHAT YOU ARE DOING – YOUR THOUGHTS AND ACTIONS		

When there is a gap between what you know to be true – your values – and what you are actually doing, you'll suffer energy draining negative emotions such as regret, depression, anger, anxiety, disillusionment, stress, aggression and fear because you are not upholding your highest truth or potential. At the most important level, not fulfilling your highest potential and not doing your very best in all areas of life is the biggest cause of being out of integrity. Described here is the biggest cause of disease in this world. Take this literally. When you are out of integrity your body loses vital energy and creates a toxic environment which is the largest cause of dis-ease in all people. When you do not uphold your highest integrity you create constant conflict in your mind where you think one way and act another way. In simpler terms, to be out of integrity is to live the lie to what you know to be true.

Whatever you do that is not aligned with your integrity will utterly drain you of all your energy and disconnect you from the whole. Your thoughts will become incessantly consumed by your ego and you will continue to feel drained. When you are out of integrity you will not have the connection to Energy required to fulfill your purpose. The negative emotions that being out of integrity brings you are all emotions that allow you to realise that you are not living to your highest potential and

---
4 Philosophers Notes

have lost connection to Universal Energy. When you are able to close that gap by living in a way that you know to be true, you become reconnected to Energy, which always brings you to feeling more vibrancy, happiness and fulfillment. Simply, to close the gap between what you know to be true and your thoughts and actions is to create a blissful life.

As you can see, when there is an integrity gap, unfavourable emotions begin to creep into one's life. Whilst these emotions that are described are quite 'negative' and undesirable, realising that they occur due to the way that one is living out of integrity is actually very positive.

Just as was described earlier, these emotions can be likened to an alarm clock making an effort to 'wake you up'. There is an obvious reason why we all get these emotions, our bodies and mind's are telling us that something is wrong. Just as becoming happy is our minds way of telling us that we are doing things well, human beings have been intelligently created to have an amazing capacity to let us know when we're off track and out of integrity. We need to learn to connect with our emotions and learn from what they are trying to tell us. The alarm starts ringing to let us know that we need to change the way we are living. You will feel so empowered when you view such 'negative' emotions with a new perspective. If you feel sorry for yourself when you experience undesirable emotions you will simply continue to live out of integrity, and thus suffer and continue living an unfulfilled life until you learn from what life is trying to teach you.

However, if you begin to view these feelings and emotions as an amazing gift that your Higher Power bestows on you to allow you to realise that you have been living out of integrity and that you have lost your connection, you will become empowered to change. So let's firstly accept these emotions as an incredible gift. You are aware that acting and living your life in certain ways can either make you feel good or bad. If you want to have a strong spiritual connection and live a constantly happy life; I cannot stress how important it is to live your life in-line with your highest integrity. This doesn't only apply to the big issues; it applies to *every* single area of your life.

I live in integrity by maintaining a certain set of daily fundamentals. My fundamentals are the things that I know help me to be at my absolute best and live my life upholding my truest values and expressing my truest self. They all connect me to Energy. I want to fulfill my purpose and fulfill my potentialities by providing the world with what I was born to give it, and to do that effectively it is imperative that I'm always at my absolute best.

Just like trees have roots that hold them steady during the most forceful winds, maintaining fundamentals allows us to ground ourselves so that we may be free to always express our truest selves, no matter how turbulent our lives become.

My daily fundamentals include:
- Meditating for 30 minutes when I wake up
- Journaling my highest virtues and values
- Exercising for at least 30 minutes every day
- Eating healthily
- Creating (this includes writing, blogging and reading)
- Giving to others
- Being present as often as possible
- Being appreciative by being grateful for everything/everyone in my life

It requires self–control to maintain these fundamentals every day, but self-discipline and self-control are like a muscle – the more you use them the stronger they get. Studies have found that if you demonstrate self-control in one area of your life, you also instantaneously develop self-control in many other areas in your life. For instance, as you muster the self-control to begin a regular exercise program, you also become much more willing to eat healthily and rest more.

I also make sure that I do not do what I know does not align with my highest integrity: gossiping, lying, blaming others, judging or taking people for granted. The activities that I have just listed are the things that I know allow me to be the absolute best person that I can be. Each activity is fully aligned with my highest integrity, allowing me to have a spiritual connection and remain present and *highly energized* all the time.

My fundamentals are so important in regards to allowing me to be the person I know will fulfill my purpose, that if someone offered to pay me $1 billion to stop doing any of the exercises I simply would not accept it. You may be thinking to yourself that my previous comment is flippant or even idiotic, but the fact remains that I know I was born into this world to fulfill my purpose, and to fulfill my purpose I know that I need to live my highest integrity and maintain a strong spiritual connection. Everything else is secondary. Not only do these activities allow me to be at my absolute best, they also bring me natural positive feelings and emotions that money can never buy. Quite simply, no amount of money is worth jeopardizing the pursuit of fulfilling my purpose and potential, and hence, living a meaningful and fulfilling life.

I know for certain that I have a strange feeling that flows through my body when I don't maintain my fundamental activities and don't live my highest integrity. I become anxious about what is going to happen in the future, I became stressed, less secure about myself, judgmental of others and I feel like something is missing in my life. Often I feel depressed when I'm consistently out of integrity. My body literally creates toxicity and I can feel tension and stress in my back and neck. Sometimes I even get a headache. Most importantly, I become completely drained of energy and am zapped of the energy required to fulfill my purpose. My creativity seems to vanish and I lose the connection with my Higher Power that is needed to fulfill my purpose effectively. I lose confidence, feel unfulfilled and crave an escape. I even start eating poorly. Do these feeling resonate with you? At this point the alarm clock is well and truly waking me up. I know for sure that I get these feelings when I'm out of integrity – whether it's from drinking too much alcohol, eating unhealthily, not exercising, doing things that harm my body or mind, doing things which I know aren't right or doing anything that I know isn't going to help me be at my very best. No matter how small my misalignment of integrity is, it always affects me in one way or another.

On the other hand, when I maintain my fundamental activities every day I literally feel connected to Energy. I release all anxiety, worry and fear which is replaced with happiness, gratitude, faith and confidence. I sense a feeling where I know that everything is going to work out fine. When I'm feeling like this, I know that I'm in my absolute best condition to give my greatest strengths in greatest service to the world. You will find that Universal Energy rewards us with guidance, strength and positive emotions when we constantly live our highest integrity and do what we know is right. If you want to achieve personal fulfillment and success you must align every aspect of your life with your purpose – that's what fundamentals are all about.

PRACTICE

- Find some paper and a pen and start journaling these questions. Feel the incredible energy and connection to Universal Energy that comes from consistently living your highest values and truths. In every single moment, always do what you know is right.

- **What daily fundamentals can you create for yourself?**

- **What do you know would benefit you that you do not currently do on a regular basis?**

- **What can you do to live your highest integrity?**

- **What disciplines can you implement into your life that will support your deepest purpose?**

- **What is one thing that you can start doing <u>right now</u> to align yourself with your highest integrity?**

- **What is one thing that you're currently doing that you can stop doing <u>right now</u> to further align yourself with your highest integrity?**

MEDITATION

If it was possible to take the benefits of meditation and put them into pill form, meditation would be the highest selling drug *ever*.

Meditation is free, has immense benefits and no side effects. Meditation literally helps you to become a better person and live a better life. Most importantly, meditation is one of the most effective methods to connect you to Universal Energy.

Modern day living causes many stresses in our lives which block our connection to Energy. Our bodies and minds are constantly working overtime and our busy lifestyles are pushing us to new limits all the time – we're always on-the-go. All over the world people are suffering from more psychological and physical illnesses than ever before because there is so much going on in our lives that drains our energy. The stresses from this state of life not only drain our current energy, they also stop our ability to efficiently renew our energy from natural sources, including from foods and exercise. Daily problems are seemingly taking a hold of people and intensifying until they become too much to handle.

Our minds are working overtime. We generally do not have any control over our thoughts, which are like drunken monkeys swinging from tree to tree. A non meditator is controlled by their thoughts and thus their ego. A meditator controls their thoughts and functions from a much more powerful source. There's a substantial difference in relation to energy. When people are controlled by their thoughts, they are limited to the energy that they can gain from natural sources, whereas those who have the ability to control their thoughts hold the ability to control their energy intake, and thus the quality of their lives.

If you want to live your happiest, most loving, most fulfilled life, it is imperative that you live in a stress-free, relaxed environment and have efficient energy flowing through you so that you may fully express your truest self. To facilitate this you need to release all built up tensions and find more ways to live blissfully, relaxed and free. Meditation is the answer.

Meditation doesn't take years to master and you certainly do not need to become a yogi or Buddhist. Meditation is one of the simplest, most natural ways to connect to Energy.

Benefits

As you begin to establish a regular practice of meditation you will wake up every morning feeling highly energised and really excited about the prospect of meditating because you simply know that it is so good for you.

Here is a summary of the benefits that you will gain as you maintain a regular practice of meditation:
- Unlimited source of natural energy
- Decreased stress, tension and anger
- Reduced fear, anxiety and worry
- Improved clarity and better decision making
- Improved calmness, peace and relaxation
- Increased happiness
- Stronger immune system functions
- Improved health and physical condition
- Increased motivation to exercise & eat healthily
- Longer, deeper, more efficient sleep
- Increased memory
- Increased self-understanding
- Increased self-confidence
- Improved relationships

As well as the ability to:
- Slow the process of aging
- Change the functions of your brain
- Create a more positive perspective
- Become non-reactive, non-resisting and accepting
- Overcome depression
- Overcome addictions
- Speak to your highest self

All of these benefits allow you to fully energise your body, mind and soul. All this – just from meditating. It is nothing short of miraculous!

As humans, we put a lot of our time and energy into looking outside ourselves for energy, love, happiness and peace, yet as you begin to meditate, you will realise that you have always had a direct link to Energy within. We also spend a lot of money trying to buy medications and other masking agents like alcohol to fix our problems and reenergise. This is precisely why meditation has become a popular alternative healing technique for people with illnesses such as cancer. Meditation allows the body to stop the flow of negative energy within and replace it with renewed, efficient, positive energy. Meditation helps you to let go of inner pollution so that you may rediscover your authentic self.

As discussed, we very rarely focus on the present moment. The majority of our thoughts and energy are spent either worrying about how events in the future are or aren't going to work out or we are thinking about things that have happened in the past that cause us guilt, failure and negativity. Meditation allows us to fully engage our energy and experience what is happening in the present moment on a deeper level. By practising to still and quieten the mind, you will train your mind so that it is capable of conducting energy. When you regularly meditate you feel emotions more fully, you laugh more, you feel more love, you develop more gratitude for the beauty around you, the energy of life flows freely through you and you create a life of consistent wellbeing – no matter what your circumstances may be.

When we increase our awareness and stop incessant 'thinking', we are able to live in the present and accept things for what they are – without judgement. When we become aware rather than judgemental, we realise that nothing is good or bad unless we give it that meaning and that we always have the power to choose how we perceive all of our circumstances. Life decides our circumstances and we are empowered to choose our response. In this sense, meditation allows us to stop feeling like a victim and become more empowered. When you uphold a consistent meditation practice you will find that the things that used to cause problems in your life simply no longer affect or hold power over you. Instead of reacting to 'problems', you accept what is happening with a sense of peacefulness and calm, no matter what happens. As a meditator, 'problems' simply will not affect you the way that they do those who do not meditate.

What Exactly Is Meditation?

Meditation is a discipline which uses advanced breathing techniques where one can train the mind to a deeper state of consciousness, leading to deeper states of relaxation and awareness.

Simply, meditation is an awareness of inner silence that allows you to focus on the present moment. Meditation is often perceived as something that is complex and hard to master, but simply, meditation is the practice of controlling your breathing and controlling your thoughts in order to control your brainwaves and thus create a heightened sense of awareness. As we control our breathing we relax, energise and unwind all of our tensions and stresses, and as we control our thoughts we open our minds to endless benefits and possibilities.

Your brain is constantly going from thought to thought. Studies have shown that we have over 50,000 thoughts per day. It is beneficial to put this into perspective. If we have 50,000 thoughts per day then we have at least one new thought every two seconds. Your mind is constantly working and without rest. When your mind is constantly bombarded with thoughts and stimuli it simply cannot operate at its highest potential and is unable to connect to the presence of Energy.

When I first began to research meditation, I read many books and on-line articles to get my head around what meditation actually is. I had heard that there were many benefits; I just didn't know how it actually worked. Then I came upon research and information about how meditation can positively affect our brainwaves. After reading about how meditation can slow our brainwaves, I was hooked and had the sudden motivation to meditate every day.

Meditation literally changes the frequency of our brain waves. The frequency of these waves lowers so that we are able to experience higher levels of consciousness, altered states of mind, connection to Energy and all of the other extreme benefits that go along with such change.

By controlling your brainwaves you can also control your state of mind, and thus your energy. Brainwaves are electrical movements in the brain. As meditation allows you to slow your brainwaves, it also allows you to have greater power over the way you act, feel and think. And by connecting to Universal Energy you can also control and strengthen your health, happiness energy levels and immune system.

The human brain functions in four different states; beta, alpha, theta and delta. As our brainwaves slow, we are able to become more relaxed. When we are awake our brains usually reside in a beta state. In a beta state our minds are most alert. We are able to analyse problems, process information, listen, think and undertake everyday activities. Whilst beta brainwaves are very beneficial in helping us to function in our day to day activities, being in a beta state too frequently can cause stress, anxiety, over thinking and limited healing time for our bodies.

The goal when you begin meditation is to change your brainwaves from a beta state to an alpha state. Alpha brainwaves allow you to feel relaxed, calm and peaceful. It is the state in which you can fully energise. In today's world many people rarely get to an alpha state due to stress, nervousness, fear and worrying. To get to an alpha state you need to slow the constant thoughts that come into your mind by relaxing and breathing deeply and practicing this on a regular basis. By doing this, you remove mind clutter and allow your brainwaves to slow into a deeply relaxed state.

When you are able to shift your mind into an alpha state you can begin to experience superior levels of energy. You are able to function more efficiently, increase performance, feel more relaxed and much less stressed and anxious. In alpha you also have better memory, better social interactions and deeper sleep. On an even deeper level, meditating in an alpha state allows you to reprogram your brain to remove negative false perceptions and bad habits caused by your ego and replace those with new positive chains of thoughts and habits. The energy sustained from this practice completely invigorates.

As you progress further into your meditation practice the goal is to shift your brainwaves from alpha to theta. In a theta state you are able to become highly creative. The world's greatest ever musicians, painters and artists experience more theta brainwaves than others. As discussed earlier, the greatest people who have ever walked on this earth were all connected spiritually to Universal Energy. These people all used their vast levels of energy to create greatness in the world. Meditation is the one of the greatest means to acquire the exact same Energy. Shifting into a theta state helps to create a spiritual connection and experience even higher states of relaxation. In a theta state you will feel more vibrantly alive and experience more positive natural emotions rather than stressed emotions. In theta you will also be able to connect with your subconscious mind, find answers to your problems and be guided by your deepest intuition. By controlling your brainwaves through meditation you can literally gain control over your life.

Meditation allows your mind to be free of thoughts that prevent you from connecting to Energy. When free of thoughts, a mind in meditation has a feeling of oneness with your Higher Power. It is believed that being in a theta state is being in complete alignment with Universal Energy. As a non meditator or a beginner to meditation, it's easy to be sceptical about this. It cannot be proven scientifically that this is the case, although you are likely to find that most meditators truly believe it. Before I began meditating, I thought that is was absurd to suggest that anyone could connect to a Higher Power just by meditating. However, as an experienced meditator, I now feel with 100% certainty that I'm strongly connected to Universal Energy every time I meditate. When your mind is quietened it creates space for your subconscious mind to communicate with you. I truly believe that this is like talking to the same Energy that created this world.

I concur with the many spiritual teachers who say that a prayer is when you talk to Universal Energy, whereas meditation is when you listen to Universal Energy. If I've ever wanted to receive an answer or guidance, my biggest life questions have always been answered whilst I was meditating. When I wanted to know what my life purpose was, I asked whilst I was meditating and I received an answer. The answers don't always come straight away but they definitely come eventually if I'm willing to persistently ask and remain consistently present.

You too can find answers and seek guidance if you are willing to show faith in this exercise. If you want to know if you're travelling on the right path or if you have other specific questions that you'd like answers to, bring yourself to a theta state and receive the guidance you require from Universal Energy. If this sounds too farfetched, don't let it deter you – meditation provides many other benefits that will enhance your energy.

Meditation is more important in today's times than ever before. We seem to be getting extra busy and extra stressed *all the time*. This leads to us often being unhappy and frustrated. These negative moods and emotions directly drain our energy which *always* leads us towards poor health. People are so busy in their day to day lives that they 'don't have the time' to stop and refuel, causing them to hold on to toxic stress. This always leads to dissatisfaction and conflict due to an unconscious need for energy. This is why it is so important that you use meditation as your energy refuelling station.

Stress is a state of physical or emotional strain that is caused when the body reacts to stimulus or situations which it perceives to be dangerous. To put it simply, you become stressed when your body (unconsciously) reacts to situations that suck your energy from you. It all relates back to our primal days when our bodies created stress as a 'fight or flight' mechanism to heighten our senses when a life or death situation occurred, such as a dangerous animal coming close by or hunting for food when the body was almost starving. Both activities take the body's natural energy. In the primal era, the small amounts of cortisol released into the body was valuable because it gave a short burst of energy that the body needed to renew strength so that it could fend off any danger.

Nowadays, we still have the same fight or flight mechanisms that cause stress, yet instead of becoming stressed once every now and then due to a 'life and death' situation such as the attack of an animal, in today's world we are stressed from life's most mundane activities *all the time*. Many things trigger our stress. You will discover that every single stress steals your energy from you; being cut off whilst driving, receiving too many phone calls, eating junk food, getting bad customer service, feeling constrained by time, receiving negative comments from a colleague or doing too many things at once. The list of things that cause us stress could go on forever. All of these little things cause us stress and accordingly our bodies are being pumped with high levels of cortisol to try to compensate for the lack of energy.

When you become stressed and low on natural energy, your body produces cortisol to heighten your awareness and help you to continue doing what you do. Over time, too much cortisol (created by too much stress and limited energy) causes your blood pressure to increases, tensions in your body and an unhealthy immune system. This then starts a vicious cycle which makes you even more stressed, which leads to more cortisol, which leads to more stress – leaving you completely drained of spiritual energy and full of toxicity. The body thinks that it is under attack and so tries to gain energy from others in any way possible.

The overload of stress is what generally causes us to get headaches, sleep poorly and constantly feel lethargic and run down. Studies[5] have shown that heightened cortisol levels will inevitably weaken our immune system and leave us susceptible to illness and disease if we don't take time to relax our body and mind and reenergise. A consistently energy deficient, stressed body is an ideal breeding ground for illnesses. It's really important to become aware of the effects that stress has on your

---

[5] Palacios R., Sugawara I. (1982).

body and mind. Just being aware will exponentially help to increase your motivation to meditate.

Unfortunately, this is a description of the life of many people. The build-up of all this stress and the toxic energy in the body is what causes illness and disease. There is little wonder our youngest generations are estimated to live shorter lives than their parents – even with better medication and more efficient technologies than ever before.

Effects of Low Energy Caused by Stress

On the body:
- Tension
- Shallow breathing
- Less oxygen in the cells and tissues, causing acidic waste products to accumulate in the body
- Acidic environment in the body
- Elevated blood pressure levels
- Elevated heart rate levels
- Higher cholesterol in the blood
- Weaker immune system (prone to diseases, infections, allergies, etc)
- Poor digestion
- Higher levels of toxins in the bloodstream
- Inability to effectively nourish, heal, or regenerate properly

On the mind:
- Excessive thinking
- Fear based thinking
- Anxiety
- Aggressiveness
- Poor communication

This is why meditation is so important. Meditation provides us with the required energy to overcome the overwhelming struggles of daily life. The oxygen which you breathe in when meditating energises and radiates the body, creating the same feeling that exercise brings. In Latin, meditation translates to *mederi*, which means 'to heal'. The natural energy that meditation provides heals the body and the mind by bringing it back to a state of vitality. More and more doctors all around the world are beginning to prescribe meditation instead of drugs to heal the symptoms of stress and anxiety. Doctors are realising that medication only treats the symptom, and although the symptom may be eradicated by medication, the patient is still left depleted of energy (which caused the illness in the first place) and is thus just as likely to continue getting more illnesses until the initial problem – the patient's energy levels – has been solved. Simply, there is no medication as powerful as that of Universal Energy gained through meditation.

Obviously, no one wants to suffer from these adverse results of stress. Meditation affects the body in the complete opposite way to which stress does by restoring tremendous levels of natural energy and making it highly beneficial for the body and mind. Meditation will help you to relax and provide you with the energy required to overcome stressful situations and stimulus that arise. As your energy renews, your body will return to a stress-free state where your blood pressure drops, your heart rate slows, your oxygen intake becomes more efficient and your immune system strengthens. This all helps to heal your body and prevent further damage caused by stress, whilst at the same time providing you with the energy to overcome any problems that you hold onto from the past. In this state, you will begin to slow down and enjoy the smallest, simplest, most beautiful things in life. Your newfound appreciation of beauty will then energise you even further.

Enhance your Energy

Best yet, as you increase your energy and reduce stress, your body is able to more efficiently allocate the resources that you give it. Your body becomes more efficient in using food for energy and allocating vitamins, nutrients and minerals to your cells. This leads to even further increased energy levels. You'll even have better quality sleep which will also lead to further energy levels. Reducing stress and increasing relaxation through meditation helps you to have a deeper delta sleep. Delta sleep is where our body can work its magic on ultimate restoration. If you've ever woken up feeling really reenergised, it's likely that you had a delta sleep. You can expect much more of that when you begin a practice of regular meditation. As you decrease stress and tension by meditating daily you'll feel invigorated, rested and bounding with energy, allowing you to bring a new sense of self to every aspect of your life and literally become a better person.

When you begin to meditate you will realise that there is much more to life than you would have ever imagined. As you begin a regular meditation practice, release the ego and begin expressing your true self you will begin to see and admire beauty everywhere you look. You will admire the amazing functions of the world, the amazing functions of the human mind and body and you will release attachments from the things which matter least.

How to Meditate

Meditation is much less complicated than you probably think. I will here provide tips to get you started meditating at the beginners level.

With first hand knowledge of how incredibly energising and life enhancing meditation is, I suggest that you try to meditate for fifteen to thirty minutes every day. My highest recommendation is that you commit to meditating **every day**. Build this habit by setting aside the same time every single day. You will see benefits from meditation if you practice it every now and then, but you will realise much more incredible benefits once you make your practice a daily habit. Challenge yourself to commit to meditating daily. You may naturally hold resistance to this idea, but know that it will likely be one of the greatest gifts you will ever give yourself. It is suggested to start meditating for just ten minutes per day and naturally progress to fifteen minutes, then twenty minutes, then twenty five minutes and eventually thrity minutes per day. Increase your time as you feel ready.

Many people believe that the best time to meditate is first thing in the morning. When you have just woken up your mind will most likely not be bombarded with as much stimulus as it would be throughout the day. It is much easier to energise when you don't have lots of different thoughts popping in and out of your mind like a drunken monkey. Morning is also the quietest time of the day. I wake up, have a long, warm shower and then go to a quiet spot to meditate. Meditating first thing in the morning also makes it much easier to maintain a daily routine, as you don't have any excuses to stop you from meditating. If you have to wake up early to go to work, you just need to wake up thirty minutes earlier. At first thought, getting up thirty minutes earlier than usual does not sound like a good idea! Worry not about fatigue, because you'll find that thirty minutes of meditation is the equivalent to many more hours of sleep. After your morning meditation session you will be feeling highly energised, calm, invigorated and ready to blissfully start the day.

Wear lose clothing and take your shoes off so that you don't feel any restrictions on your body. This will allow a free flow of energy around your body.

Always try to clear you mind before you begin. If you meditate first thing in the morning, this should not be a worry. If you meditate throughout the day or at night time, it is likely that you will have lots of different thoughts running through your mind. Try to release these thoughts by writing them down before you start. If you have things to plan out or to do after meditating, write them down on a piece of paper. Alternatively, do whatever you can to relax. Take a shower, have a bath, read a book or go for a walk and then find a quiet spot to sit and meditate. For ultimate benefits, it is really important to meditate in an area free of disruptions. Find a quiet spot where you will feel comfortable, warm and able to relax. Play some calming music or light a candle to set the mood if you feel like it. This is your time to relax and reenergise.

When you think about someone meditating, you probably picture a Buddhist monk sitting in a yogi position with their legs crossed. This is widely thought to be the ultimate position to meditate in, allowing the most efficient flow of energy throughout the body; however, it is not the only way to meditate. The yogi position requires great flexibility, making it unrealistic for most people.

When meditating you can sit however you want, as long as your back is straight and you are comfortable. Your back must be straight in order to have a maximised flow of energy throughout the body. Sit in a chair in an upright position if sitting on the floor in a cross-legged position is too uncomfortable for you. If you cannot sit upright in a chair for whatever reason, you can alternatively lie flat on your back on the floor – just make sure you don't fall asleep!

Allow your hands to relax into your lap or on your knees. Relax your face and mouth.

I recommend that you keep your eyes closed lightly and relaxed. If you find it too difficult to concentrate with your eyes closed, find a picture or object to concentrate on with your eyes open until you feel comfortable about keeping your eyes closed.

Relax

Start each session with several power breaths. Emphasise the breath as if you were about to blow out the candles on your birthday cake, then push it all out until your lungs are empty. Breathe in until your lungs are full, and release again. Do this several times to enter new oxygen and energy into your body and to release old energy.

Relax your body by sending your attention to each body part. Focus your attention on your feet and feel them relaxing into the ground. Feel your bottom relaxing into the ground or your seat. Feel your hands relax into your lap. Scan all of your body parts from head to toe and feel your entire body begin to relax as you take several emphasised breaths. Feel your heartbeat begin to slow.

It is likely that you will feel tension in one or more areas when you begin meditation. This is because you aren't used to sitting and concentrating in this position. Direct energy towards any areas of your body that are feeling tension. Breathe in and mentally direct your oxygen towards any areas of tension. It is a great thing that you feel this tension – it is negative energy that has come to the surface because it wants to release itself from your body. Feel the new energy entering and flushing the tension away. Relax. Feel the peacefulness.

Breathing is a really important part of meditation. Deep breathing relaxes the muscles, slows the heart rate and helps the mind to focus. It also brings new oxygen into the body which energises each and every cell. During everyday life we are not mindful of our breathing and hence breathe shallowly. Generally the only times that we breathe deeply are during exercise and laughter. Did you ever wonder why you feel so great when you exercise and when you laugh? Just as when you meditate, serotonin (the happy hormone) is released into your body plus you breathe deeply, bringing plenty of fresh oxygen into your lungs. Fresh oxygen circulates to flush new energy throughout your body. The power of oxygen is amazing, highly purposeful and highly energising.

Meditation is about concentrating on your breath so that you can still your mind, decrease stress and allow your body to reenergise. When you begin meditation you might notice that you have hundreds of different thoughts that float through your mind. The goal of meditation is to not give any attention to these thoughts. Simply accept that they are there, push them aside and continue to always focus on your breath. It will be beneficial for you to know that every single person who meditates has lots of different thoughts passing through their mind during every session – this is natural. Do not think that you are not meditating correctly if you have lots of thoughts going through your mind. It happens to everyone – allow yourself to relax and feel the deep peace that comes from your breath.

It's recommended that you breathe through your nose to allow the greatest flow of oxygen to reach your brain. If this is difficult for any reason, e.g. if you have a blocked nose, breathe through your mouth.

The most popular breathing method for beginners is to count your breath. Counting your breath puts further attention towards your breath so that your mind doesn't wander off with your thoughts.

When you inhale, say 'one' in your mind, and repeat 'one' again during the exhale. Inhale again and repeat 'two', then again when you exhale. Continue this method until you reach 'ten' and then count your way back down to one. This can be continued for as long as you feel comfortable. If you lose count, start at one again.

Always focus on your breath – this is what centres you in the present moment. Start by noticing and feeling the breath in and the breath out. As you progress into your meditation, feel the breath as it enters your lungs and fills your body. Feel how it fills you with new energy every time you take a new breath. Feel the new energy reaching each and every part of your body. Feel your renewed and reenergised body relaxing into your seat. Feel your body relax and release tension as you exhale. Feel the absence of breath when you have fully emptied your lungs. Feel any old, unwanted energy leaving your body. Feel the stillness and peace. Feel that each breath is taking you to a higher state of inner awareness and connection with Universal Energy. Feel the deep happiness and contentment that comes with every breath you take. If your mind wanders away from focusing on your breath, re-establish contact and focus on the breath again.

What Should I Meditate About?

The greatest reason for meditating is to release negative energy, connect to the unlimited source of Universal Energy and align yourself with the purpose of your life. Personally, I find greatest relaxation and energy comes to me when I consciously try to meditate about nothing and remain fully present to my breath. My sole focus is on clearing my mind and focusing on my breath the entire time. I still have many thoughts floating through my mind. My aim is to be aware of these thoughts, not give them my attention and continue to focus on my breath. By meditating like this, I am able to remove all of the clutter from my mind, be aware of the thoughts that I have, de-stress, ponder nothingness and reenergise. It might not sound very appealing, but 30 minutes of stillness and quietness (especially in today's chaotic world where we are always nonstop) has amazing relaxation and energising benefits. The emotions that I feel after meditating like this are almost indescribable. If you're a busy person who is always on-the-go, you will find that this type of meditation has the ability to lead you towards a really relaxed and invigorated state.

As described, I have asked many deep life questions and always received answers during and after meditating. The process of meditation quietens your ego, allowing you to discover yourself truly. Sometimes it takes time to receive an answer, but as I persistently ask the things that I want to know, the answers always come. Over time I have asked and received answers to these questions:

- **What are my greatest passions?**
- **What are my greatest strengths?**
- **How can I use my passions/strengths in service to the world?**
- **How can I get paid to give my passions/strengths in service to the world?**
- **What is my purpose?**
- **Am I currently on the right path?**
- **How can I best align with my purpose?**

It often takes time, but the answers always come. You will instinctively know when you receive an answer because you will have a feeling of oneness with the soul of the world.

PRACTICE
Here is a guided meditation based on the information above:

- Find a quiet spot where you will feel comfortable, warm and able to relax

- Sit in a position that allows you to have you spine straight so that you feel comfortable

- Relax you mind and body. Relax your feet. Relax your hands. Relax you torso. Relax your bottom. Relax your face. Feel the relaxation as you body sinks into your seat

- Take several power breaths

- Feel your heart beat begin to slow down

- Breathe through your nose. Focus on your breath

- Feel your breath fill your body. Feel the new energy beginning to flow through you

- Exhale slowly and feel the old energy leaving your body

- Concentrate on your breath. Take deep and full breaths

- Begin counting each breath as you inhale and exhale

- Inhale 'One'

- Exhale 'One'

- Feel each breath brining you further into peace and relaxation. Feel each breath bringing you into a higher state of awareness and connecting you with Universal Energy

- Continue counting until you reach ten and then count backwards

- Notice thoughts coming into your mind. Accept that they are there, and allow them to pass by without any more of your attention. Return your focus to your breath. Always focus on your breath

- Feel your breath filling your body. Feel the new energy flushing through your entire body. Inhale. Exhale

Continue this practice for as long as you feel comfortable. This is all you need to do to begin meditating. It is not as hard as you may have thought. Don't stress or worry if you feel like you are not meditating correctly. Like all good things, the practice of meditation can take time to develop. Keep persisting, because the benefits are definitely worth it. You may be thinking to yourself 'Is that it? Are you sure that's proper meditation? I thought meditation would be much harder than that?' It is that simple. You now know how to meditate. All you need to do next is take action.

GRATITUDE

One of the easiest and most effective ways to connect with and gain tremendous energy from your Higher Power is to be grateful for everything in your life – to appreciate your life, the people in your life, the possessions that you have and even the world itself. It is *impossible* to be grateful and depressed at the same time. Scientists have proven that those who express gratitude for their lives are much more likely to be happier than those who are not grateful. Research conducted by Dr Robert Emmons at the University of California-Davis found that people who kept a journal and wrote down five things that they were grateful for every day enjoyed increased happiness, increased energy levels, were more optimistic, felt healthier and even exercised more frequently than those in a control group who did not keep a gratitude journal. Dr Emmons found that people who make a conscious effort to appreciate their life are also more likely to help others, be less materialistic, more spiritual and are much less likely to suffer from depression, anxiety and jealousy.

Have you ever noticed that when you buy something new, for instance a new car, you seem to see that car everywhere you go? The brain has an area called the reticular activating systems (RAS) which brings the things which you place importance on to your attention. If the brain did not have a RAS your mind would have to work in a frenzy to process all of the information that surrounds you. When you're walking through a busy shopping mall your RAS is what allows you to block out all of the noises and people and allows you to focus only what you place importance on. Oblivious to most people is the fact that we can deliberately program our RAS to only process information which we deem to be important. In regards to everyday life, most people don't consciously program their minds and instead unconsciously give their greatest energy to things which strengthen the ego, for instance things that they can complain about. As this is what they place greatest importance on, the RAS continues to find more things for one to complain about. However, by consistently being grateful for everything in your life, you can train your RAS to only find things which make you grateful. Just like you seem to see other people driving the same car every time you go for a drive, your mind will allow you to find things which make you grateful and happy.

By training your brain to find things to be grateful for, you bring more and more things into your life to make you happy, even if your outside world doesn't change.

This creates an incredible cycle where you find more and more things to be grateful for, creating a consistent connection with Universal Energy and feeling tremendous energy freely flowing though you. It's simply logic; think about what you appreciate and what makes you happy as frequently as you can and you will be rewarded with incredible energy and more reasons to be happy.

Having an 'attitude of gratitude' is incredibly energising and one of the simplest ways to connect to your Higher Power. It doesn't matter what you are grateful for, whether it be the clothes on your back, your friends or family, the plants in your garden, the food that you eat or a smile that someone gave you, being grateful energises you, making you feel deeply blissful, happy and vibrant. It is impossible to feel unhappy when you truly appreciate the things in your life. Gratitude allows abundant energy to flow into your life as you become aware of the greatness of your life and all that you have in the *present*. Wishing, wanting or hoping for things in the future brings anxiety and fear, whereas being grateful in this moment, no matter how much or how little you have, brings joy and positive energy.

Universal Energy has created every single thing in your life, from the food you eat, to the air you breathe, to you, to the world you live in. When you are grateful for your life and everything in it, your Higher Power rewards you with energy for your appreciation. As you appreciate, your energy increases and you gain an immediate feeling of connection with everything that surrounds you. By appreciating Universal Energy for all of its creations you generate a sense of oneness with every person and every aspect of your life. Appreciating the people and things in your life reminds you that everything is connected, that you are alive for a specific purpose and that you are not alone in this world, allowing you consistently to find meaning and to enjoy the present moment. Gratitude is the bond that unites us all.

On the other hand, if you are not grateful for what has been created for you, you are not going to get any favours or energy from your Creator. New Thought writer Wallace D. Wattles says, *"You cannot exercise* much power without gratitude; for it is gratitude that keeps you connected with Power." In fact, it is highly likely that you will feel alone, disconnected and become narcissistic in an effort to gain energy from others if you do not appreciate the life that you have been blessed with.

Just sitting here, I am so thankful to have a computer to write this book, the internet to educate myself and connect with many people and the publishers and distributors who got this book to you. I'm grateful for the beautiful house that I live in that provides me with comforts, warmth and shelter. I'm grateful to have access to running water, I'm grateful for the sun that keeps me warm, electricity that powers all of the *amazing* technologies that I have, the food I just ate which gives me incredible energy and I'm grateful for my family and friends - I could go on forever. Even just thinking about how incredible the human mind and body is and the way that we function gets me really excited. Being grateful for these things makes me feel light, peaceful and blessed with the knowledge that I really do have everything that I need to live a great life. Gratitude for these things makes me feel deeply connected to Universal Energy, and I know that I will continue to gain even more things to be grateful for as long as I am connected to this Energy.

Sometimes it's easy to find things to complain about and take the little things that I was just describing for granted – but it is just as easy to find things to be grateful for. For example, my power went out at one stage whilst I was writing this book. Life gave me two options; I could have complained that I had no electricity and consequently felt really negative about it, or, I could have been thankful that I even had power in the first place. After all, 200 years ago electricity didn't even exist! People certainly didn't have central heating to keep them warm in the winter or the luxury of a power outlet to charge their computer, because computers weren't even conceived of back then. Life gave me the choice to either complain about my situation, or choose to use it as an empowering experience which would intensify my appreciation for the world we live in.

Think about your own life. Do you get upset when the traffic is bad? What a great opportunity to marvel in the wonder that the world is so advanced that you even have a car and can travel to a destination in air conditioned comfort. Do you get angry when your telephone company gives you poor service? What a great opportunity to quietly thank Universal Energy for creating such an incredible technology that allows you to talk to people from all over the world through a *piece of plastic*. Do you get annoyed when restaurant waiters are rude to you? What a great reminder of how you would like to communicate with people. What a great opportunity to appreciate the fact that you can afford to eat out. Appreciate that you can even communicate with others.

It is just as easy to let everyday events drain your energy and create a negative mood as it is to see that these situations give you the opportunity to be genuinely grateful for all of the amazing things in your life. Within every aspect or area of your life lies something for you to get excited about. Be grateful for the little things - many people living in this world do not have the same luxuries as you.

If you choose to take the negative perspective of any situation, you will inevitably feel grumpy, stressed, anxious and completely drained of energy. Worst of all, if you incline your mind towards things that you're unhappy about, your mind will continue to find even more things to make you unhappy. If you instead chose to have an 'attitude of gratitude' and look to really appreciate how lucky you are to even have certain 'problems' in your life, you are going to feel empowered, happy, full of energy and blessed to be alive!

So if you want to gain consistent energy, happiness and fulfillment, look for things to be grateful in every moment of your life. I highly recommend that you journal about everything that you are grateful for at least once per week. When you wake up, make a mental list of all the things that you're grateful for – this is one of the greatest ways to begin your day highly energised and ready to give your purpose to the world. Brian Johnson says, *"If you get pissy/impatient while sitting in traffic, definitely look to alchemize that energy into some more positive. Perhaps each time an impulse to curse the traffic arises you can mentally run through all the people you have to thank for even having the opportunity to be stuck in traffic when it wasn't too long ago you would've been on a horse... and the last time I checked they didn't have AC. Send silent appreciations as you imagine the person who sold you the car, the people who put it together, the people who created each piece before they got assembled, the people who worked with the raw materials, the people who made the street you're driving on, and, perhaps, you can give a shout out to the Big Guy in the Sky who made ALL THAT?!?"*

Meditating about what you're grateful for is another incredible way to connect to Universal Energy. Meditate about all of the great things in your life that you truly appreciate.

Another empowering exercise is to meditate about all of the things that you're unhappy with in your life and see how you can turn them around to be things to be grateful for. You now know that everything happens for a reason, so how about appreciating all of the challenges and 'tougher' times that you have encountered throughout your life. These events have shaped your life – you wouldn't be who you are right now if none of these things had ever happened and every single one of these events has led you towards your purpose – so be grateful for them! If 'bad' things happen throughout your day, thank them for teaching you a new lesson. You can find ways to be grateful for absolutely everything that happens in your life. If someone is rude to you quietly be grateful for them reminding you how you *don't* want to act. By being grateful for the things that don't quite go the way you would have hoped you are in effect saying to Universal Energy, 'I trust in the path and purpose that you have given me.' Hidden beneath all things that don't go your way lie lessons that you *need* to grow.

With this perspective you can incline your mind so that it is constantly looking to find great things in your life, rather than 'bad' things. Best yet, as you appreciate all the greatness in your life and realise how blessed you really are, you become much more inclined to give to others; and giving will always increase and intensify your energy.

Beauty can be found everywhere you look. The whole world is beauty. Let's quit complaining and make a conscious decision to look for all the amazing things in our lives and be thankful for them. Let's not forget how blessed and fortunate we are to have everything in our lives, including life itself. Let's not take the little things for granted. Know that more will come to you if you enjoy what you've already got rather than wishing for more or thinking that you'll be happy/satisfied when you receive more. And don't forget, you would not have anything in your life without the service and help of others. You wouldn't even have the chair that you sit in whilst reading this book if it wasn't for the service of others. Without the interconnected web of service from others you would not survive. We are all connected. Be grateful for every person and absolutely everything in your life – you will be amazed at how energized, excited and happy you will feel when you adopt an attitude of gratitude.

So what are you grateful for? How can you put more energy into being grateful in your daily life?

PRACTICE

- It is highly recommended that you journal what you are grateful for at least once per week. This has scientifically been proven to boost happiness levels. Grab a pen and journal *everything* in your life that you appreciate.

- Think about what you appreciate and what makes you happy as frequently as you can. Have the intention to notice everything good that happens to you. With any spare moment that you have, make a mental list of all of the things that you are grateful for.

- Don't take the little things for granted.

- Knowing that everything happens for a reason, turn any 'negative' circumstances into an opportunity to be grateful. If 'bad' things happen throughout your day, thank them for teaching you a new lesson.

LOVE WHAT YOU DO

All of the people who have ever grown a successful business, achieved noteworthy achievement or made a vast difference in this world loved what they did. By loving what they did they were able to draw the vast Energy that is required to achieve anything of noteworthy success. If you want to achieve meaningful success it is imperative that you love what you do. All of the great thinkers and authors agree that following your bliss and doing what you love is vitally important.

Many people say, 'Life is short'. I disagree. Life is impermanent and time limited, but it is also extremely long! If you live for 80 years – that's a really long time. If you are going to live for such a long time, you must create quality in your life by doing what you love. Loving what you do every day gives you incredible energy and allows you to feel vibrant and radiantly alive. When you do what you really love to do you will have unlimited levels of enthusiasm. The happiest people to walk this world are those who discover their greatest passions and figure out a way to fully align themselves with doing what they love every day.

Considering that you spend more time at work that any other area of your life, the most defining choice that you may make in your life in terms of your overall happiness and energy is to love your work or find work that you love.

Take a moment to think about what you truly love most in your life. Whether your greatest love be music, sport, food, travelling or anything else, think about how high your energy and happiness levels would be if you did that thing that you love every single day. Let your imagination run wild.

No doubt, your life would be incredible! You would enjoy amazing levels of energy, bliss and fulfillment *every single day*. Well, I am here to tell you that this great life is not limited merely to your imagination. Each and every single person on this earth loves what they love *for a reason*. A person's greatest love and passion is strongly aligned with *what they are meant to do*. This is why 'knowing thyself' is the greatest knowledge that one will ever gain in their lifetime. It is so important that you know what you love so that you can invest the majority of your energy into doing it as much as you possibly can. When you do what you love you are in full alignment with Universal Energy. I can say without any doubt whatsoever that your life will be full of joy, meaning, fulfillment, energy and bliss when you design your life so that you consistently fulfill your greatest love in alignment with your purpose.

On the contrary, not loving your job and 'just getting through' the day so that you can go home at night and 'just get through the week' so that you can enjoy your weekend is a depressing and unfulfilling way to live. Working to 'pay the bills' or to 'earn a living' creates conflict in your world because the very fact that you aren't fulfilling your potential goes against your integrity, creating a little voice in your head constantly telling you that you can do better. If you spend your life being a doctor whilst deep down you desire to be a musician, you will live a conflicted, frustrating and miserable life. The majority of the moments that you spend doing work because 'you have to' sucks your energy, leaving you feeling empty, dissatisfied, disconnected and full of toxic energy.

It saddens me to think about all the people in this world who are working a job that they do not like. They spend the majority of their lives doing what they really do not want to do, feeling unhappy and powerless. Some of these people think that there is no other option other than to work this job that they dislike and they lack the courage to change their circumstances. We all know people like this. You may even be a person who does not like their job. Think of friends or family members who are constantly complaining about their jobs. Rather than choosing their current jobs because they are passionate about a particular field, it is most likely that they have chosen these jobs based on extrinsic motivations. These motivations include money, status, recognition and other benefits. Many people do not care what profession they are in as long as they are earning good money. Little do they know that their Higher Power has much greater plans for them.

In regards to your work and the job you do, your emotional and physical energy are determined by your source of motivation. If you are primarily motivated extrinsically by secondary benefits such as money, status, recognition or other benefits, you will go through the motions and be drained of energy because you know that there is a contradiction of integrity between what you are doing and what you know you are capable of doing. Neglecting your unique gifts and the reason for your creation creates a disconnection between yourself and Universal Energy.

Whereas, if you are motivated intrinsically and do your work because you love it, feel that you are contributing yourself to a greater cause and gain intrinsic fulfillment and satisfaction from it, your life will prosper and bound with energy.

Sourcing your motivation intrinsically also ensures that you are more likely to maintain the self-discipline, integrity and persistence needed to achieve your goals because the success of your goals is determined by your own level of satisfaction as opposed to the satisfaction of others.

If you find yourself constantly fatigued, dissatisfied, complaining or stressing about your job, or if you don't like your co-workers, your working conditions, or the actual job itself, know that *you have the power* to change your circumstances.

Once you have found your purpose you will discover that it is highly viable for you to do work that you absolutely love. You will love your purpose so much in fact that you'd be willing to do it for free. After all, your intelligent Higher Power created you for this purpose.

If you want to live an incredible life you must learn what gets your juices flowing. Now that you've completed the activities to discover your true self, your energy must be placed into designing your life so that you only do the things you love. Not loving your job drains your vital energy and happiness, meanwhile, loving your job fills you will incredibly vibrant energy, happiness and fulfillment. It is within your power to create a life where you constantly do what you love. Do not waste your life doing things that you do not love and certainly do not get to your deathbed and regret that you never fulfilled your potential. You have been uniquely created for a specific reason – fulfill that reason.

PRACTICE
- Avoid doing anything because you *have* to as much as possible. Do everything because you *love* to. Create your life so that your work provides meaning and care to the soul of the world. Personally, I'm not willing to do work that I don't love in order to gain secondary benefits. I know that my life is much wealthier when I follow my purpose and what I truly love and that the secondary rewards will eventually come anyway. It is completely within your power and choice whether you are willing to do things that you do not love.

- If you feel like it is not possible to create a change to doing what you love, continue doing what you're currently doing and incline your attitude and perspective so that instead of doing your work because you 'have to', you find reasons to *love* what you currently do. Find ways to bring joy and love to the things which you must do. Look for the great aspects – the things that you are grateful for – in your current job. It may be easier than you think. Most importantly, discover your purpose; it will guarantee that you *love* what you do every single day for the rest of your life.

LOVE YOUR UNIQUE SELF

Loving yourself is so important that it cannot be overstated. Loving yourself is directly linked with fulfilling your purpose and living a life of happiness, love and fulfillment. Every time that you don't fully express who you truly are your soul shrinks a little bit. Ultimate happiness comes from embracing your uniqueness and giving yourself to the world.

Your true self is free of ego. It is free of false self-image, free from fear of criticism, free from a fear-based need for approval, thus allowing you to fully express yourself. The more you admire and love yourself, the more energy you can give to and receive from others. Being in a consistent state of love will give you an infinite amount of energy – so much that it doesn't matter how much others take from you. If you fully love, accept and appreciate the person who you are, you are *guaranteed* to live a happy life.

Regardless of what you think of yourself, the truth is that you are a unique, divinely beautiful person. To deny yourself this truth is to deny yourself of an incredible life. If you don't currently love yourself, or if there are aspects that you do not like about yourself that you think others judge, now is the time to change. Your opinion of yourself very much determines the person who you show up as in your life. If you do not love yourself you must fail to realise that each and every person past and present has been created for a specific purpose. Everyone is created uniquely divine so that they can fulfill that purpose and be the person that they were created to be. To compare yourself to others is the work of the ego. When you stop comparing yourself to others and fully embrace and *love* everything about yourself, you will undoubtedly live an incredible life.

Embrace Your Uniqueness

Whilst we know that everyone is connected and alike, we also know for sure that no two people have ever been created the same. Every single person on this planet has unique fingerprints, personalities and appearances. Even 'identical' twins have different characteristics and mannerisms. We are all created to be unique and to express our true selves. Understanding your uniqueness is fundamental to finding the meaning of your life. Universal Energy never has and never will create any human, animal or plant to be exactly the same as another. This being the case, ask yourself if you are trying to be like others.

You are created to express your unique individuality. There is nothing wrong with you – anything that you think is a negative aspect about yourself is really only something that is specially unique about you. To compare yourself to others is to shrink your soul. **Every single person has purposefully been created to express their unique gifts.**

We are all meant to be different – there is no doubt about it. If we were all meant to be the same, we would have been created to look the same, have the same mannerisms, enjoy the same hobbies and do the same things. Wouldn't that be boring?! Many people fail to see that they have been created uniquely and have a bright light within them that is waiting to be shone upon this great world. People think that something is 'wrong' with them, when the thing that they think is 'wrong' with them is really an expression of their uniqueness and individuality – it is what's special about them.

You must embrace your uniqueness. Any aspects or characteristics of yourself that you see as liabilities are really just part of the divine, perfect you; embrace those things about yourself.

The failure of people to see their true potential and purpose drives them towards trying to fit in with everyone else. You know how it is – everyone wants to wear the same brands, drive the same cars and go for the same jobs. By following the collective you shrivel the true you; the divinely created, purposeful soul. Rather than 'getting rid' of the qualities that you dislike about yourself, it is so important that you find the *positive* aspects of these characteristics and embrace them into your life.

People lack the courage to be different, which is perplexing, because *we are all different in the first place*. To be like another is to be compelled to the egoic mind. The very word 'identification' derives from the Latin words *idem* and *facere* which translate to 'same' and 'make' – to make the same. So identifying to certain products, jobs and ways of being is really the ego's way of trying to be like everyone else because it has fears that you will be seen as a 'nobody'. Without really knowing it, when you buy a designer label or car you are not so much buying a product, but something to enhance your identity. But, as discussed, the ego is never satisfied – it always wants more. It always wants to impress and make itself feel like a 'somebody' no matter what you acquire.

Have the possessions that you own and the amount of money you make become part of your identity? Have the clothes you wear, the car you drive and the house you live in become part of who you are? Have these 'things' slowly become more important than love, compassion, enjoyment and living a life with meaning?

Do you try to use 'things' to enhance who you are? If this is the case for you, your life is being controlled by your ego rather than your true self. We find ourselves trying to identify our lives by attaching ourselves to that which we think will impress others. But nothing is ever good enough, so we keep pushing for the next thing to identify with, and then the next, and so on. This is a great way to feel depressed because with every pursuit to impress others you create a bigger integrity gap and drift away from fulfilling your greatest potential and shining your truest self upon the world.

If you want to live an extraordinary life, you need to overcome the ego by having the courage express your uniqueness. Be willing to be *you*. We all look different and we all act differently, and it doesn't stop there. We all have our own unique purpose on Earth – we each have a specific mission that we have been born to achieve.

If you lack the courage to shine your unique light, you'll settle with following the status quo and end up criticizing those who dare to be different. When you fully love yourself you will never blame, criticize, gossip or put others down. Why? Because you only do those things as a way of making yourself feel bigger and better than others to satisfy the ego. When you fully love and accept yourself, there is no need to put yourself on a pedestal.

Once you love yourself you won't feel a need to abuse yourself or others. You won't need to put others down and you certainly won't feel the need to put yourself down. If you currently abuse your body and mind with substances such as alcohol, drugs or over eating, *loving yourself* will end your desires to 'escape' through such measures by connecting you with Universal Energy and filling the void that previously you've been trying to mask.

Deep within every single person though, nobody wants to live a mediocre life. We all want to make an impact and stand for something. Deep within everyone lies grand desires and aspirations to create greatness with our lives. We all want to make a difference. Yet, what sets those who make a difference apart from those who live mediocre lives is the amount of courage that one is willing to bestow in order to express one's unique self. Everyone fears failure and the potential judgements that come with it. But the lack of courage and fear that one feels is not the truth, it is not real; this is simply a deep fear of the ego. The ego fears the judgement from everyone that will occur if you fail. However, you will gain the courage to express your unique self when you become spiritually inclined and eradicate the false 'sense of self' that the ego creates.

Be willing to be vulnerable

Be willing to start pushing your comfort zone and being *you*. When you make yourself vulnerable in the judgemental eyes of others you actually give these people the power and confidence to live their highest truth too. I was once walking along a highly populated beach listening to music on my iPod. When my favourite song started playing I really felt like singing it out loud, but my ego overpowered me and told me that everyone else walking along the beach would think that I looked ridiculously silly. So I stopped singing. I chose to let the judgement of others smother my true self, until I became presently conscious. I questioned myself; 'What do I have to fear? That I will look silly? That I will embarrass myself?' Suddenly I thought, '*Who cares!*' I replaced the negative expectation of the idea that others would think that I looked silly to a positive expectation – that I could really enjoy myself. I started singing softly and as my confidence grew I started to really sing quite loudly – and it felt great! I realised that by putting ourselves in 'vulnerable' situations like this we are each able to help others to also think, 'You know what, I'm going to be myself and do more of what I want to do and not allow myself to be restricted by what society wants me to be like'.

If you truly want to live the life that you are meant to live, be prepared to look different, act different and be different to others, including your family, your friends and your community – and love the person who you are. The freedom that comes from expressing your true self is incredible.

You have so much energy to give the world. Be prepared to put the energy into finding your passions, strengths and purpose and then give it to the world, no matter whom you think will judge you.

You have been created with specific gifts and talents. These gifts are given to you so that you may fulfill your purpose, your mission, your destiny. This is not an egotistical drive to be better than everybody else; it's simply a fact that you are a unique person and you have unique gifts to give to the world. This is an incredible realization and one that you should fully embrace. You weren't born into this world to live the status quo or to shrink your soul by fitting in with the mediocrity of others; you are here to shine your unique self and create greatness with your life. We weren't all created differently so that we could end up being the same. We weren't given unique strengths, values and passions so that we could fit in with what everyone else does. We weren't all given a specific purpose so that we could neglect it and work towards our own egoic goals. So come on, push your boundaries, embrace your uniqueness, love who you are and follow that deep drive within you to be different.

You must begin at once to *love yourself* exactly as you are – divine, unique, beautiful and purposeful. If you think you're ugly – you're not. If you think you're a 'nobody' – you're not. If you think others are better than you – they're not. If you think that you're worthless, know that you are worthy of anything you want. If you recognise yourself in any of the aforementioned traits, your-self judgement only comes from what 'society' thinks, which is generally a shallow collective egoic delusion anyhow. You are the beautiful manifestation of Universal Energy. The same Energy that created the beautiful mountains and oceans of the world also created you.

No matter what you look like, no matter your personality, no matter what others think of you, *you were created to be the way you are for a specific reason* – what a beautiful thought. The world needs you, and it needs you to realise that you are an amazing person.

The Platinum Rule

The commandment known as the 'Golden Rule' states that you should treat others as you would like others to treat you. I like that rule because it provides a guideline that one treats others with respect and loving kindness. However, I much prefer Tal Ben Shahar's version of the golden rule, which he calls the 'Platinum Rule'. The Platinum Rule is to *"Treat yourself the way you'd like others to treat you."* The Platinum Rule accounts for the way that you treat yourself, which I believe is far more important than the way that you treat others, because inevitably the way that you treat yourself determines the way that you treat others. Most people treat *others* better than they treat *themselves*, which is quite perplexing. Many people would never judge, speak harshly to or put others down, yet they do these exact things to themselves all the time. Many people disrespect and treat themselves unkindly, creating within a dissatisfying, unhappy existence.

One can only love others to the extent that they love themselves, which is why loving oneself is of primary importance to loving others. By fully embracing and accepting yourself, and thus treating yourself with respect and loving kindness, you will form a connection to Universal Energy that will dramatically *improve* all aspects of your life. When you fully love and appreciate yourself, not only will you create an amazing relationship with yourself, you'll also improve your relationships with every person who you come into contact with.

On the other hand, lack of love for oneself is one of the major causes for ALL of the problems in the world from depression to disease. Louise Hay, one of the world's most profound and successful psychologists and author of the best-selling book *You Can Heal Your Life*, says, "*When people come to me with a problem, I don't care what it is — poor health, lack of money, unfulfilling relationships, or stifled creativity, there is only one thing I ever work on, and that is loving the self. I find that as we really love and accept and approve of ourselves exactly as we are, then everything in life works. It's as if little miracles are everywhere. Our health improves, we attract more money, our relationships become much more fulfilling, and we begin to express ourselves in creatively fulfilling ways. All this seems to happen without even trying.*"

Lack of self love, self acceptance and self approval is the root of nearly all of the problems that you will ever suffer from throughout your life. Insecurity, lack of self esteem and a negative attitude toward the self all cause dramatic problems in the lives of those who have not yet discovered that they are amazing, divine, unique, beautiful beings. As long as you neglect these facts, you will continue to suffer. It is worth repeating the thoughts of Louise Hay; 'I find that as we really love and accept and *approve of ourselves exactly as we are*, then everything in life works.' This is a powerful statement which must be taken literally.

To fully love yourself is to wholly accept and appreciate every attribute of your being. As discussed in the topic of gratitude, when you accept and appreciate anything in your life, you are in fact connecting with Universal Energy by showing gratitude for your divine creation. It's like you're saying, 'I fully accept, love and am thankful to be the person who I am'. There is no room for self judgement, deficient self esteem and all problems that stem from a lack of self love when you truly and wholly accept and love who you are. To love yourself is to appreciate the amazing creation that you are and to realise that you are connected to the Energy that created everything around you.

Conversely, when you don't love yourself, are not happy with and resist being the person that you have been divinely created as, you are (unconsciously) resonating energy back to your Higher Power that is saying that you are ungrateful and unappreciative for the very Energy that created you. In this state of self resistance you are fully disconnected from the great Power that created you, and thus you will encounter many problems throughout your lifetime.

Being unhappy with the world that you live in, the people who surround you or even your life situations is a clear sign that you lack *love for yourself*. When things seem to be negative in your life, for example, the weather's bad, your partner or friends are being rude to you or your job is not satisfying you, these are all examples of the fact that you are running low on self love. Have you ever noticed how the rain can make some people unhappy whilst it can make other's dance with joy? Have you ever noticed how when the weather is cold or wet certain people always make a remark such as, 'What a disgusting day'? The fact is, how you see the world is a reflection of the way you view yourself.

The world doesn't need to get 'better' – it is already divinely perfect – just as you are. The only thing that needs to change is your perception of yourself!

I didn't love who I was for a long time and there were a number of things about myself that I wasn't happy about. The world around me seemed like a dull place to live and I wasn't excited about the prospect of living a long future. Self-doubt and worried thoughts of others' judgement stopped me from expressing my authentic self, which in itself created many problems ranging from self-esteem issues to deep unhappiness. Reminiscing the times when I didn't love myself I can remember how I was unhappy with my body shape, I felt uncomfortable around others and was emotionally unintelligent. Not loving myself, it was impossible for me to fully love others, and likewise, for others to fully love me, thus I was rude to others and my relationships were non authentic. My life was mediocre at best.

Nowadays, I love myself, I fully accept and embrace all parts of my being and I authentically express myself to the world every single day. I can tell you first-hand exactly how life-changing the benefits of fully embracing and loving oneself are. I still live in the same world with the exact same conditions as previously, but my perception of the world is *completely different*. Everywhere I go, everywhere I look, I'm amazed by beauty. I can't walk down the street without feeling a deep satisfaction to be such a divine being who is fully expressing his uniqueness and purpose to the world. I've also found that by fully accepting and approving of myself, I have no need to judge, blame, criticize or be rude to others. By fully accepting myself, I'm now able to accept everyone else and appreciate their own uniqueness. I love everyone in this world just as much as I love myself.

Let me tell you that making the shift from not loving oneself to fully loving oneself is much easier than you may believe. All you need to do is accept that you have been created the way you are for a specific reason and trust that if the same Energy that uniquely created you also created this magnificent world, it definitely has great plans for you! Fully align yourself with Energy and you will see a new world. Louise Hay is one of the world's greatest psychologists. She believes that it is so important that her clients love themselves that she makes them look at themselves in a mirror and has them say the affirmation *'I love and accept myself exactly as I am'* until they say it so many times that their minds starts to believe what they're saying. Realise that you are a divine creation. If you want to live an extraordinary life, it is so important that you love your uniqueness and fully embrace everything about yourself. Stop playing the roles that society wants you to play, stop trying to fit in with others and *be yourself*. Love absolutely everything about yourself.

Another way to develop self love is to determine the qualities that you 'dislike' about yourself and begin at once to fully embrace them and fully except every part of who you are, because there is a reason that you are this person. Be willing to accept every single part of your being, even the things that you aren't so happy with. Don't deny or suppress any aspect of yourself. Become aware of who you are and fully accept that person. Rather than trying to be something that you're not, embrace what makes you different from and sets you apart from others. Spiritual Guru Osho says, *"Drop the idea of becoming someone, because you are already a masterpiece. You cannot be improved. You have only to come to it, to know it, to realize it."*

If you want to be like another, you are missing the point of your existence. Ralph Waldo Emerson says, *"Envy is ignorance, imitation is suicide."* Take those words literally. To envy, imitate, compare or want to be like someone else shows that you are ignorant of your own unique beauty and the gifts that you've been blessed with. When you neglect your own unique beauty you are not only disconnecting from the most important Energy, you are also unconsciously creating an unhappy life.

The only time that you judge or condemn yourself is when you compare who you are to others. Comparing yourself to others is a symptom of the egoic mind. You wouldn't consider yourself 'good' or 'bad' if you had nothing to compare to – you would simply be *you*.

What would you do if you knew nobody would judge you?
Who cares about what others think. Trying to be somebody other than who you are is a waste of your potential. You are not what others think of you. You are not your body. Don't limit yourself. You are a soul – a divinely created unique being. Embrace who you are!

You will discover that **your happiness will increase** immensely when you stop comparing yourself to others. **BE YOU**! Love who you are! Express your true self! It's incredibly hard to be what others want you to be, yet incredibly easy to simply be yourself. Don't try to be something that you're not. You hold incredible potential – don't accept anything less than the fullest expression of who you are. Discover who you truly are, and then express that person to the world and **don't hold back.**

PRACTICE
- Create an amazing relationship with yourself by embracing every unique aspect of what makes you who you are. What are some of your aspects that you consider 'liabilities'? What do you dislike about yourself? Uncover, own, embrace and fully accept every aspect of what makes you who you are. You are *meant* to be unique.

- If you truly want to live the life that you are *meant* to live, be prepared to look different, act differently and be different to others. Stop playing the role that society wants you to play. Stop comparing yourself to others. Be willing to start pushing your comfort zone and being you. Be willing to be vulnerable. Follow the deep drive within you to be different.

CONNECT TO SERVICE

You now know that you were made to be unique and that you have your own set of passions, strengths and values. Surely Universal Energy wouldn't create you to be different to others and give a unique set of gifts and skills so that you could live a life of egoic pleasures.

Your unique gifts were given to you so that you could fulfill your purpose, give to others and create a positive impact on other people's lives. Those who function from their deeper Being make such an incredible impact on this world. You're not here to take, you are here to give.

One of the greatest things that you will possibly ever learn is that the quality of your life is not determined by what you can get, but rather, the quality of your life is determined by what you can give. You have been blessed with a unique set of skills, passions, strengths and values to give to the world.

People all around the world want more money and work more and more hours but never seem to get anywhere. Their focus is on what they can get rather than what they can give. Once you shift your focus from 'what can I get' to 'what can I *give*' you will find an amazing change of energy in your life. You'll begin to feel connected to others and realize that we are all linked in this life together. You will see that you can make a genuine difference and create value in the lives of others. This is by far the greatest way to add meaning to your life as well as the life of others.

The meaning that you have been looking for has nothing to do with what you can get in your lifetime; meaning is found in what you can *give*. By giving to others through a service that uses the great gifts that you have been blessed with you create a strong connection to Universal Energy which is far greater than anything else that can ever satisfy your body/mind/ego and that flows abundance, meaning and fulfillment into your life.

Rather than focusing on how much you can make, gain or receive in your life, focus on what you can give and prosperity will reach you in ways that you would have never imagined. We've already discussed how the spiritual person knows that they come into this world with nothing material and that they leave with nothing material when they die. Acquire as much as you want during your lifetime, but know that the quality of your life will be determined by what you *give* to others.

Ask yourself, **if there was no money in this world, how would I best serve humanity?** You will find that as you provide your greatest self in order to fulfill the needs of others, you will naturally receive boundless wealth from many sources.

CONNECTING WITH OTHERS THROUGH GIVING

The laws of Universal Energy ensure that you simply cannot *get* anything without first *giving*. This law applies to all areas of life. Think of anything that you could ever want, from the tangible to the intangible; money, food, water, clothes, possessions, attention, kindness and love. To gain any of these things, you first need to give something. This rule of life has been created for a reason; to create a great sense of connectedness between all people. But somehow society has lost its sight of this highly important wisdom.

You would have heard the saying 'it is in giving that we receive' over a hundred times. When you do something kind for someone, your brain naturally releases serotonin (the 'happy hormone' that pharmaceutical companies stimulate with anti-depressant drugs) which literally energises you and makes you feel great. Better still, the receiver of the act of giving also has serotonin released in their brain, plus any person who watches the act of giving also has serotonin released, creating an extremely calming, happy and healthy environment. I have a strong belief that the production of serotonin is Universal Energy's way of rewarding us for creating a connection between others. Just as negative emotions symbolise an alarm clock that allows us to 'wake up' and change the way that we are behaving, serotonin is produced to remind us that what we are currently doing is what we should continue to do. This is how giving works at a biological level, but I'm certain that there is more to it at a spiritual level. Spiritually, the reason one receives from giving to another is because giving connects the giver's energy field to the receiver's energy field, exactly the same as what happens when two people begin an intimate relationship.

Whereas acting selfishly disconnects us from others (hence the creation of negative feelings created by the body when we are selfish), giving literally connects us with others (hence the amazing positive emotions we feel when we give to others). All things created by Universal Energy are energetic beings that have a soul and a potential to connect with all other souls. Giving is the connecter. I've discovered from many years of experience of selfishness that the greatest way to make myself become stressed and anxious is to focus on myself and what I can get from the world. I have also come to learn that the greatest way to feel happy, loved, fulfilled and live a meaningful life is to connect to the whole by giving my greatest self to others. It is clearly evident that giving connects us to others whereas selfishness disconnects us from others. Without any doubts whatsoever, the greatest happiness and fulfillment that you will ever have in your life will come from connecting with others, and giving is one of the greatest ways to connect.

Whenever you give to someone, externally you may give a present, love, warmth, a smile, a listening ear or whatever, but underlying these things is the gift of Energy. As you give your Energy to another, your Energy fields combine, giving you both the energy of two people. Have you ever been given a hug when you've been feeling low? When someone hugs you, they share their energy with you which instantaneously energises you and makes you feel better. Being so energised makes you feel amazing not just for the receiver, but also for the giver, and this is the reason why it is in giving that we receive.

Mastermind groups are a perfect example of the power that lies within connecting to others. A mastermind group is generally a group of four to six people who gather to discuss a common shared goal. Just the same as two batteries put together provides more power than two singular batteries operating individually, mastermind groups of people *always* produce more and better results than each person would individually. Why? When the energy fields of all people come together, each individual has the power and energy of many people flowing through them that allows each member to intensify each other's creativity, wisdom, knowledge and connection to Universal Energy. If you've never been part of a mastermind group, you may have experienced what I'm talking about when you were stuck on an idea and asked a friend for advice. Often, as soon as you ask someone for advice, (even without the other person saying a word) you create clarity in your mind because you share their energy. Unlimited potential lies within connecting energy with others.

When I was younger I came across this quote by Hip-Hop mogul come philosopher Russell Simmons: *"In my opinion, his problem was that every* day, he was waking up trying to figure out what he can get, instead of waking up trying to figure out what he can give"

The quote absorbed my thoughts for about half an hour as I re-read it about twenty times. At the time I was travelling through India after just completing a Bachelor of Business majoring in Entrepreneurship. I'd spent my whole life trying to figure out how I could make 100 million bucks. From the time that I was fourteen I'd been reading the Financial Review, Business Review Weekly and whatever business books I could get my hands on. Every morning I would wake up thinking about what I could get from the world. I wanted lots of money and I wanted it quickly. This quote hit me like a brick in the head as I suddenly realised that I had I been driven by greed, fear and selfishness for the past ten or more years.

I realised that if the quality of my life was going to be determined by what I could *get*, I was likely to live an awfully meaningless life. After all, I came into this world with nothing material and I would most certainly leave this world with nothing material. This being the case, the quality of my life would not be determined by what I could get, but rather by what I could **GIVE** to others.

I can assure you with great certainty that your life will become extraordinary if you wake up every morning trying to figure out powerful ways to give yourself to the world. Give as much energy as you possibly can to the world with the knowledge that giving to others will also enhance your own energy, creating incredible fulfillment in your life.

You don't need to give in a big way, simply start by making it your aim to give in some way to every single person you come into contact with. Whenever you meet with someone, give them love, warmth, appreciation, affection, a smile, a hug, you presence, a listening ear or a shoulder to lean on. It doesn't matter how you give, just *give*. Give positive energy. Praise more. Find the good in people. You have absolutely nothing to lose by praising someone and you will most likely brighten their day. You've got nothing to lose by smiling at each person that you walk past. Be empathetic. Give joy. Connect. You literally have the power to enhance other people's lives, and of course, your own life.

Look to create a connection and bond with others with every opportunity that you have. Every person that surrounds you is Universal Energy's unique expression. Connect with the miraculous. Smile at every person you see. Become one with the Energy of the world. Bring out the best energy in others – doing so will bring out the best energy in you – and is the surest way to improve the life of yourself and others. Give to others even if you don't feel very energised and your connection to the person you give to will automatically energise you. Even give to people who your ego 'doesn't like'. The reason that such people do things that you don't like is because they are low on energy and are behaving in a particular way in an effort to gain energy. By giving to others you bring them consciousness and reduce the power of their egos. If you give to someone and thus energise them, they will behave in a way which is harmonious and conscious. You literally have the power to create harmonious relationships even with the people whom you've never previously got on well with.

Every time someone asks you to give something to them, Universal Energy is testing you. It is testing your attitude and life perspective. If you give, it shows that you are aware of the rule of energy, that what you give you shall receive in spades. Everyone always wishes for more. Well maybe you are constantly being given the opportunity to have more every single time someone begs from you or asks you for something. Maybe when you heed these calls you will get all that you wish for in return.

Give others what they need – on a micro and macro level. Every time you give of yourself you are not only helping to add more meaning to the lives of others, your life is becoming more meaningful and you are slowly but surely creating a better world. Most of all, enjoy giving to others and creating a meaningful connection between yourself other human beings. Can you just imagine how incredible the world would be if we all transcended our egos and energised each other by constantly giving of ourselves?!

PRACTICE
- Every moment provides you with an opportunity to fully give yourself. You don't have to start a charity to fully give of yourself; you can give to others simply by smiling, being present when others talk

to you, giving praise, sending someone a message to tell them that you appreciate them or helping those who seem down. Realise that the quality of your life is determined not by what you acquire, but what you can *give*.

- Aim to do at least one good deed every single day.

Would you like to do a good deed right now?
Jump online and visit **www.kiva.org**. **Kiva** is a not-for-profit micro financing organization that lends money to those who are unable to borrow money from conventional financial institutions. They are literally changing the world by raising money in an effort to help the world's working poor make great strides towards economic independence.

Kiva envisions a world where all people – even in the most remote areas of the globe – hold the power to create opportunity for themselves and others. They provide safe, affordable access to capital to those in need to help people create better lives for their families.

The thing that I most like about Kiva is that you don't just donate your money, you lend it to an individual or group, who then uses these funds for business or educational purposes, and then they repay you. Once you have been repaid you can then continue this magnificent cycle by choosing to lend again. With as little as $25 I've been able to help a mother of four to set up a food store in Togo, a mother of eleven children to set up a nursery business in Congo, and a group of men to start a business in Sierra Leone. I've also been able to help various people in Mongolia, Peru, Nigeria and Ghana.

Kiva.org was born from the following beliefs:
- People are by nature generous, and will help others if given the opportunity to do so in a transparent, accountable way.
- The poor are highly motivated and can be very successful when given an opportunity.
- By connecting people we can create relationships which exceed beyond financial transactions, and build a global community expressing support and encouragement of one another.

Kiva.org democratizes philanthropy, allowing the average individual to feel like a mini-Bill Gates by building a portfolio of investments in world businesses. It's an incredible feeling to know that you're helping so many people who without help would be stuck to the traps of poverty.

You can help change the world yourself. Give it a try and see how good you feel!

CONNECT TO NATURE

The same Energy that created the sun, the moon, the mountains, the forests, the sea, trees, plants and other vegetation also created and runs through you. Nature is Universal Energy's expression of pure potentiality – discovering this allows us to realise that we ourselves are also an expression of pure potential. Connect with nature as frequently as you possibly can. Head out into nature and immerse yourself in its beauty as often as you can. Sense the energy that radiates from such beauty. Breathe in the crisp oxygen, soak in the sun, the gardens and the nature that has been created *for* you. Immerse yourself in the beauty of birds that fly above you. Connect with the beautiful colours of the trees, plants and flowers that have been gifted to you.

The sun is one of the greatest natural energisers. Bask in its beauty. Soak in the beauty of a sunrise or sunset. The feelings gained when viewing a sunrise or sunset flow vibrancy right through your body. These two times of the day intensely energise you and make you feel *alive*. Tremendous energy can be found by immersing yourself in nature, and it's free, easily accessible and all around you. Look for beauty everywhere; in the smile of a young child, in a tree blowing in the breeze, in the sun shining upon a field of grass. Look and you shall find beauty surrounding you everywhere you go. This beauty is an expression of Universal Energy – the same beauty lies within you.

EAT HEALTHILY

Eating healthily is highly important if you want to feel consistently energised. Food provides a large percentage of our physical energy, and the foods that you choose to eat determine the quality of your ability to feel happy, healthy and fulfilled. It is imperative that you gain the highest quality energy from the highest quality of nutrition if you are to fulfill your highest potential. You need to remember that the specific purpose of food is to provide you with the required energy to live optimally and regenerate optimally with high quality energy.

There is no specific diet that you need to follow to gain energy, you simply need to align yourself with Universal Energy by eating only the foods that have naturally been created for you. Next time you shop for food, take a close look at the amazing colours and shapes of all the marvellous foods, particularly fruits and vegetables that benefit us most. The sole purpose of these incredible foods is to provide us with the required energy needed to sustain us and hence fulfill our potential.

Depending on what goes into our mouths, eating can either energise or de-energise. Digestion is a high energy consuming activity. For example, think about how tired you feel after you eat a big meal. Many cultures take a siesta after they eat because they need to re-energise even though the purpose of eating is to energise, not to eat so much that it de-energises you. For ideal energy levels that allow you to live your highest potential, it is imperative that you eat foods that take minimal energy to digest.

The foods that give us the greatest, most vibrant energy are called high net gain foods because they give us lots of energy without needing much energy for digestion. These foods include all natural foods, but specifically, fruits, vegetables, nuts and grains. These foods are also high in nutritional density, providing extremely high levels of minerals and vitamins which energise the body from the inside out. They also provide limited stress on the body, allowing the body to gain the absolute highest nutrition. Animal products such as meat, poultry and dairy are not recommended because they are low net gain foods, requiring lots of energy for digestion thus putting unneeded stresses on the body. Overindulging and eating too much at any one time is also de-energising. Aim to eat just enough to keep you energised until your next meal. Amazingly, you will find that the more healthily you eat, the less sleep you will need. This is because as you reduce foods that are hard for your body to break down from your diet, your body is less stressed, and simply needs less rest to optimally recover.

Always remember this when you are choosing what to eat; natural foods have specifically been created for us to eat so that we can gain energy. Be in tune with nature. Eat to renew yourself with great energy and you will not only feel great, you will lose weight without having to try. In fact, eating only foods that enhance your energy levels is *the best* way to lose weight, become healthy and heal the body. After all, any food that is unnatural or processed is not *meant* for you to eat. All that you need to eat can be found naturally. Connect with your food – be present and grateful every time that you eat. Eat highly energetic raw foods, lots of fruits and vegetables and as many dark leafy green vegetables as often as you possibly can. These foods provide you with the greatest amount of natural energy and connect you with Universal Energy.

Always remember that your body is constantly regenerating, and your appearance is based on every bit of food that enters your mouth. Give your body great fuel for it to use to regenerate your cells.

EXERCISE

I'm probably just confirming what you already know here; exercise is an incredible way to energise. When you exercise, your body is filled with vast amounts of oxygen (new energy) which replaces any old or toxic energy. I cannot think of anybody I know who doesn't feel great after they exercise.

Every time you exercise you effectively renew your body with fresh energy. As discussed earlier, your body is always renewing itself with the energy that you supply it with. When you exercise, you completely renew and reenergise your entire body, allowing yourself to function at a much higher vibration. When you exercise you speed up the process of renewing your cells – literally replacing stagnant, toxic energy with highly energised vibrant energy.

As with all of the other activities, exercise allows you to become present. If you're ever feeling stressed or tired from a tough day at work, there is no better feeling that going for a run, clearing your mind and renewing it with fresh, vibrant energy.

The thing that I most love about exercise is that the brain produces serotonin (the happy hormone that is produced every time we laugh or give to others) every time we exercise, which is simply our Creator's way of rewarding us and reminding us that exercise is an activity that humans are *meant to do*. I always feel *alive* every time I exercise. I have no doubt that exercising aligns us with Universal Energy, and it certainly allows us to get our body and mind into optimal shape so that we can fulfill our highest potential. When you are fit and healthy, you have more energy to give to others, can handle *all* situations better and are simply a better person to be around.

Aim to exercise every single day. It doesn't matter what type of exercise you do, just get moving in an attempt to renew your body with fresh energy. Exercising doesn't necessarily mean that you have to run five miles or go to the gym. Do whatever you enjoy – as long as it gets your body moving. Dance, stroll through nature – just get that body of yours moving. The more oxygen you get pumping through your body, thus the harder you exercise and the more you push yourself, the greater you will feel.

Exercises such as tai chi, qi qong and yoga are also recommended for those who want to still their mind and further connect with Universal Energy.

BREATHE DEEPLY

Of course, breathing is something that your body does naturally and that you don't consciously need to do, yet unfortunately this causes a lot of people to breathe inefficiently. Mostly, we often breathe too shallowly and infrequently. Every time you can remember, take a few deep breaths. Breathe deeply as often as you can remember and you will literally feel your energy levels improve. Focusing on your breath also brings you back to the present moment. When you regularly breathe frequently and deeply you will feel buoyant, light and highly energised.

CHAPTER SUMMARY

- Your life will become magical when you begin to connect to Universal Energy.

- Live your highest integrity, be grateful, learn to love yourself and all that you do, be present, give to others, meditate, exercise, eat healthily, breathe deeply and connect to nature as often as you possibly can. Align yourself with the life that you were created for.

- Above all else, make sure that you always do anything that is an expression of your true self. Sing, dance, laugh – don't take life so seriously! Your ability to achieve happiness, love, success, fulfillment and meaning is endless when you are constantly connected to Universal Energy.

- If any of these activities resonate with you, decide what is important for you along your journey of growth and commit to it integrating some or all of them into your life every single day.

How to Overcome Obstacles Along Your Journey

Only one thing will stop you from fulfilling your purpose: the often overwhelming fear of failure, which brings with it the potential feelings of shame, vulnerability and disconnection from others. Only one thing will allow you to overcome fear: the *courage* to be vulnerable. To be courageous is to be willing to be imperfect, which is perfect in itself. To be courageous is to tell the story of your life with your whole heart. To be courageous is to be compassionate to yourself by allowing your authentic self to shine upon the world. Anything less is not an expression of your highest potential. A willingness to be vulnerable creates guaranteed power, growth and beauty. What makes you vulnerable makes you beautiful. To be vulnerable is to be alive, energised and on purpose.

It's highly likely that you may need to make changes to your career and lifestyle to bring your purpose to life. Usually the thought of doing such a thing would seem crazy, maybe even impossible. But you know that this is the right thing to do. You know this is what you were born to do – you know that Universal Energy has got it all sorted out for you. Besides, you can never really fail if you're continually learning new things that are bringing you closer to fulfilling your potential.

Once you know your purpose, only one thing is going to stop you from fulfilling it: *fear*. Fear is an ego created limitation of the mind – **fears seldom become reality**. If you feel afraid to fulfill your purpose for whatever reason, know that your ego is the only force behind that feeling. The ego always tries to stop us from doing things that it knows are good for us. It tells us things like, 'You don't need to exercise today', 'You've been good today... you deserve some chocolate', and 'You don't need to meditate today, sleep in for a bit longer'. When you finally find the courage to change your life situation, your ego is the little voice in your head that says, 'Well I suppose my current lifestyle isn't that bad.

Maybe I could give it another six months to see if things can improve'. The ego knows that your growth creates the ego's decline, thus it tries to stop you from doing things that it knows will benefit your growth. Your ego will automatically try to hold you back because it fears many things. It fears that you will fail, it fears that you might succeed beyond comprehension, it fears criticism from others, it fears that you will waste your time and amount to nothing. Your ego fears that even the smallest mistakes could make you look worthless. These feelings of fear are the natural feelings that everyone has when they are about to embark on a life changing journey.

The more fear that you feel to do something, the greater probability that thing is certain to provide growth towards the evolution of your soul. If it wasn't going to provide growth to you, why would your ego have any reason to make you fearful? Don't allow the ego to stop you from becoming who you were born to be.

By far, the biggest fear you will endure is the fear of failure. In today's culture nearly everybody fears failure, so much so that the fear of failure stops many people from taking the first step. I want you to know that **failure is not bad**. As I discussed earlier, there is no such thing as 'bad' when you are spiritual. To fulfill your purpose, you have to be willing to take a leap and step through any fear of failure that you may hold. Conquerors share the same level of fear as cowards, yet what sets conquerors apart from cowards is the way that they respond to fear. The people who have achieved the greatest things in this world have all had a good relationship with failure.

There is no such thing as failure

If you want to live an amazing life you need to create a positive relationship with failure. In fact, create the mental position that **there is no such thing as failure**. There is no such thing as suffering and there is no such thing as failure – nothing is ever wrong – other than our interpretation of events. With the great knowledge that everything is purposeful and happens for a reasons, remind yourself that fear is simply *false evidence appearing real*. Failure helps us to grow. If you do 'fail' in your attempt to fulfill your purpose, you will learn many lessons to help you along your journey. When you are spiritually connected and believe that everything happens for a reason, nothing can ever go wrong. If you 'fail', that failure is *meant* to happen to help you grow towards a higher potential that allows you to fulfill your purpose. Failure is simply a nudge in the right direction. The only failure you can ever make is not taking any action. As you move through your fears, you will realise that your fear of failure is actually *worse* than any actual failure itself.

You must be aware that any fear that you feel is simply a dis-ease of the ego. You must also be aware and accepting that the fear you feel is simply what the ego uses to establish a sense of identity for itself. If you are unable to see the fear as an illusion of the ego it will quickly cripple you by causing self doubt, insecurity, anxiety, and completely diminished confidence.

If you want to fulfill your purpose, your reason for being, it is imperative that you don't allow the mind made delusions of fear and self-doubt stop you from achieving amazing results in your life.

Have the courage to overcome your fear. There is no doubt that you're going to need to be courageous if you want to live an extraordinary life. You may need to take risks, you may need to feel uncomfortable at times, but it is all well and truly worth it. Gain the courage to live the life that *you are meant to live*. The truth is that the process that you have to undertake in order to fulfill your purpose is a path that the greatest people in this world have shown is possible. Those who have walked before you have shown that the path is smooth and easy to take once you find the initial courage. Just like when you know that you should go for a run and the weather is cold and wet, the hardest part is getting yourself going. The easiest thing to do is to think about all of the excuses and reasons why you shouldn't do it, yet once you take the courageous leap to leave your current situation and get out onto your path, after warming up, the rest is then easy, smooth sailing. Besides, finding the courage to take risks will allow your life to be highly interesting. Your world will become exhilarating when you set yourself a challenge that has the potential to dramatically improve your life.

Be willing to fail - to fail means to have tried, to try and fail means to grow, to grow means to become better and stronger. Learn to accept your fear, see it for what it is, and push forward knowing that as you move through your fears you are going to grow exponentially.

Knowing that fear is simply a state of mind, motivate yourself with the thought that you are in total control of your mind, thus you are in total control of your fears. As long as you control your mind, how you control your fear is *your choice*. Preparing your mind to accept fear is going to dramatically help you to overcome it, but before anything can happen, **you must be willing to take action.**

Abraham Maslow says: *"It seems that the necessary thing to do is not to fear mistakes, to plunge in, to do the best that one can, hoping to learn enough from blunders to correct them eventually."*

Action *always* overcomes fear. Any feelings associated with fear such as anxiety, tension, stress and worry are all caused from being too focused on the future. When you begin taking action, the past and future dissolve, and you are left with a great tool – focus on the present. When you focus on the present, there simply are no problems and the past and future are merely misguided imaginations of your mind. Whatever you are afraid of will diminish as soon as you begin taking action. Create positive expectations in your mind and take the leap of faith. If you always do what you are afraid to do the cessation of fear is always certain.

Feel the fear – then make the choice to either step back into safety or step forward into growth. If you step back into safety and don't take any action the fear will fertilize and increase to the point where it becomes impossible for your mind to believe that you can take action. As long as you procrastinate and sustain from taking action, your fear will continue to intensify. You will feel fear, anxiety, stress and disillusionment when you are not doing what you know you should be doing – that is when you are not in integrity. The 'negative' feelings such as fear and anxiety are actually very positive because they have been produced by your body to tell you that you're off track. The negative feelings are like an alarm clock that is trying to wake you up and help you to realize that you need to make a change. Universal Energy knows that by not taking action you are not fulfilling your potential. If the alarm clock wakes you up, you can accept the fear and step forward into growth by taking action. Your life will become more and more extraordinary as you demonstrate this kind of real courage. You will feel great when you constantly do what you know you should be doing and your life will improve out of sight when you start taking action and stepping forward into growth.

Fear is imaginary – it's simply a negative expectation. When you fear a certain thing, you expect that something is going to go wrong.

You will have fear as long as you continue to think about how wrong things could go. But if you can change that negative expectation around to a positive expectation you'll begin to see how everything can go *right*. Let's apply this to the biggest human fear – the fear of public speaking. People fear public speaking because they are worried about all the things that could go wrong. 'I might say something stupid', 'I will look like an idiot up there', 'What if I forget what I'm going to say and freeze on the stage. I'll look stupid'. These common thoughts are all negative expectations. The best public speakers have positive expectations and confidence that they will do well. They think about how easy the process of public speaking is. Instead of thinking about what might go wrong, they think about what will go right. Change your negative expectation into a positive expectation and your fear will be replaced with confidence and enthusiasm.

For those who fear the criticism of their friends and family, you must constantly remind yourself that following your purpose is your divine right; it is what you are *meant* to do. Don't let your fear of a negative expectation regarding what other's may think about you stop you from doing the one thing that will allow you to live an incredible life. It doesn't matter what others say or think about you; what matters is what you say to yourself. If you know that what you're doing is the right thing to do, follows the guidance of your heart and is your purpose in life, the judgment of others shouldn't even come close to affecting you. As long as you fear criticism from others you won't be able to *fully express your true self to the world* – perhaps the most important method of living a fulfilling life. You are specifically and purposefully created to be unique; do not shy away from your divine beauty. Be willing to be vulnerable.

Those who make themselves vulnerable to the opinions and judgements of others are the ones who *always* create positive change in the world. Think about this statement carefully. If you follow your purpose you will have to do things that make you vulnerable to the opinion of others. You'll have to buck the trend in one way or another, and that will always evoke judgement from others. Yet, judgement from others only comes due to their egos which fear that your courage to follow your purpose will make them look cowardly. Close your mind from any negative or discouraging influences and continue to uphold faith in the Energy that surrounds you knowing that following your purpose is the correct path to travel. Stoic Philosopher, Lucius Annaeus Seneca once said, *"If you shape your life according to nature, you will never be poor, if according to people's opinions, you will never be rich."* Don't let others steal your energy from you. Continue to fully love and embrace the person who you are.

Once you are able to maintain a positive relationship with fear, the most powerful quality that you can ever acquire in order to squash your fear is a burning desire to fulfill your purpose. The energy created from having a burning desire is so strong and so intense that whilst you maintain it fear will quickly run into the corner and hide.

If you find yourself still feeling fearful about any areas of your life, take confidence from this amazing and very truthful quote of Paulo Coelho; *"The fear of suffering is worse than suffering itself. And no heart has ever suffered in search of its dreams."*

Having 'realistic' expectations

On the quest to fulfill your purpose it is wise to have 'realistic' expectations for your journey. I dislike the word 'realistic' because it creates a limiting perspective, but you can't expect that everything is going to go perfectly to plan on your quest to fulfill your greatest potentialities. Your quest to fulfilling your purpose and potential is a journey, not a destination. By fulfilling your purpose, you will inevitably create greatness, meaning, fulfillment and satisfaction within your life, but you can't expect that there won't be some setbacks along the way. All of the people that you admire and respect went through their own level of challenges, just as you will have to. Along your journey you will embark on a number of setbacks, obstacles and will probably make many mis-takes. Once you are able to accept the fact that you will have setbacks on your journey, you will then be ready to start creating excellence.

It is unlikely that you will build an institution overnight along your quest. Be willing to put in the work over the long term, knowing that the journey and present moment is just as important as the end goal. This may mean that you have to do some sort of part time work to support yourself whilst you work towards creating something of value. The world needs more people who are willing to show the way and lead by example in fulfilling their potential – even if it means that they have to do other meaningless work in the mean time. People who have the courage to do this show the world the importance of persistence, patience, passion, strength and an unwillingness to give up. You too can show the world that anyone can take a leap of courage to immerse their lives in what they love. Nothing great ever comes overnight. You *will* create greatness and find deep meaning in all that you do if you put quality time into fulfilling your potential.

You are bound to make many mistakes on your journey to fulfill your purpose, but you must know – there is *nothing* wrong with making mistakes. Of course you are going to make some mistakes in the process of **transforming your life**!! Every mistake or failure is a great thing, as it helps you to learn and grow.

Thomas Edison failed 10,000 times in his efforts to invent the light bulb. He said, *"I have not failed. I've just found 10,000 ways that won't work."* Edison knew that *everything happens for a reason* and that every failure brings with it the seed of an equivalent success. Nearly every person who has ever achieved anything great throughout history has had to endure moments of defeat and failure – it is a strange and magnificent truth of life that sets apart people of average success from people of great success.

Napoleon Hill studied over five hundred of the world's most successful people and said, *"If the first plan which you adopt does not work successfully, replace it with a new plan; if this new plan fails to work, replace it in turn with still another, and so on, until you find a plan which does work. Right here is the point at which the majority of men meet with failure, because of their lack of persistence in creating new plans to take the place of those which fail."*

Just like a baby does when it learns to walk, you're going to fall down countless times when you work towards creating anything of value. Babies don't have an internal dialogue every time they fall down saying 'You idiot! Why did you fall over again? Imagine what everyone is going to think of you. You're such a failure. You can never do anything right.' Instead, babies fall down and then get right up and try again. They stand and fall, stand and fall, stand and fall over and over again until they finally learn how to walk. Babies hold the blue print for creating anything in life. When you fall down, get straight back up again. Never give up, disregard what others may think about your fall, continue to persist and you can achieve anything.

The journey to fulfill your purpose becomes so much more fun and playful when you simply stop allowing mis-takes and setbacks that come your way to affect you. You know that everything happens for a reason, allowing you to have a positive perspective every time you fail. Falling down and struggling to overcome challenges is never a bad thing – it simply helps you to grow one step closer towards personal success.

There is no doubt that along your journey obstacles will get in your way. Remain self-assured with the knowledge that if you maintain patience, persistence, passion and playfulness at times when you come across obstacles, mis-takes and plateaus, you *will* fulfill your purpose.

You know that nothing great has ever been created without persistence, diligence and patience. The same applies for your life. To fulfill your purpose, you're going to need to work for it. Make a 100% commitment to wholly immerse yourself to fulfilling your purpose and you will find that the harder you work, the luckier you get.

Persistence

Persistence is perhaps the most important quality that you need to maintain if you desire to live an incredible life by fulfilling your purpose.

Persistence is a state of mind that you're going to need to uphold to push through all obstacles, including the obstacles that you create in your own mind. It is unlikely to expect that you will fulfill your purpose straight away. It could take months or years. You may even devote your entire life to it. Don't let this put you off. Persistence is easy to maintain when one has a burning desire to achieve any noteworthy goal. In this case, you goal is to fulfill your purpose. Your desire is to fulfill *the purpose of your existence* and live a highly happy, loving and meaningful life. One will never hold higher desires, thus, you will find it easy to remain persistent for as long as you maintain that desire.

Align yourself and connect with as much natural energy as you possibly can and know that you have the power to achieve anything that you wish for as long as you your are connected with Universal Energy. It's as though your Higher Power notices your persistence and rewards you for it.

A funny fact of life is that meaningful success is never acquired without having to really prove that you want to achieve it. It's as though your Higher Power will test you to see how much you want to achieve the goal of fulfilling your purpose. This same Energy that created this world will always reward you for your persistence and courage.

No matter how much you want to fulfill your purpose, nothing will ever be a substitute for persistence – nothing can replace its importance. You need to be persistent, especially when you seem to be making slow progress. Success will *always* come to you if you maintain steadfast persistence. Anyone who has ever achieved noteworthy, lasting success will tell you that persistence is the kryptonite to failure and success would not have been possible without this quality.

Create plans for how you will align yourself with fulfilling your purpose and then follow those plans persistently with stubbornness so that you will not stop trying until you fulfill your unique mission on earth. Remind yourself every day by writing in your journal that you are highly persistent and will not stop until you have seen your goal through.

Be patient

When fulfilling your purpose, you need to have solid patience and persistence and realise that the journey of fulfilling your purpose is just as important, if not more, than the end goal that you are trying to reach. There is no need to drop everything that you're currently doing to begin fulfilling your purpose. The key is to be patient. In today's society we are so used to watching movies, TV shows and commercials where people take up a practice and see results straight away. We're conditioned to think that something should work straight away, and if it doesn't we generally quit. Be patient and enjoy the process. Enjoying the process is far more important than the end goal that you are trying to obtain.

Let go of expectations and remind yourself that fulfilling your purpose is the best thing that you can ever do in your life. Know that just like everything else in the world, you have been created for a specific purpose and that you will progress towards fulfilling it as long as you are patient and persistent.

Rather than becoming overwhelmed by the entirety of your purpose, aim to make patient progress through baby steps. Start small and gain momentum. Don't let yourself become overwhelmed by 'big' goals. The repetition of small successes leads to greater success, and if you make many small successes you will eventually bring yourself to the point where you are doing things with ease that you never thought you were capable of.

Knowing that everything happens for a reason, trust that when things don't seem to go your way that there is a higher reason, a grander plan that Universal Energy is manifesting for you. The easiest thing for anyone to do when they come across temporary defeat is quit. The majority of people living in this world quit when things get a little bit tough. Quitting is easy, yet not an option for the spiritual person. To quit is to return to a meaningless life, whilst to fight through such obstacles is to fulfill your potential and create greatness with your life. Always trust that the whole world is conspiring in your favour.

Happy Journey!

You've done enough reading. *Now* is the time to create greatness in your life.

You've been blessed with incredible gifts. Now is the time to give them to the world. Planning and thinking about what you're going to do will only take you so far. Make a leap and begin taking action. Take risks and crush your comfort zone. Whatever you do, don't remain doing nothing. Begin your quest now. Fully express all that you feel within. Take the first step, then the next, and so on.

Embrace all uncertainty. You may encounter uncertain times on your journey of purpose. You must trust that the longer you able to embrace uncertainty, the closer you will come to fulfilling your purpose. You've taken the leap of faith, you know your purpose, now you must be willing to embrace uncertainty. And remember, life would be very boring if you always knew what was going to happen. Embracing uncertainty is your road to freedom. The longer you are able to embrace uncertainty, the closer you will be to creating greatness.

Be at your best. To ensure that you remain in integrity and effectively give your greatest self in greatest service to the world, you need to be in peak mental and physical condition. Connect to Universal Energy. You need to be at your best. Look after yourself – eat healthily, exercise, rest, and don't abuse your body or mind. Read, give, love, appreciate and create beauty for the world.

Remember that the extent of the benefits that you receive is wholly dependent on the level of commitment that you are willing to put in. As long as your internal dialogue is 'How can I help?' and 'What can I give?', Universal Energy will always look after you. Now is the time to create the life of your dreams, to fulfill your potential and shine your light brightly, proudly and playfully upon the world. Now is the time to start living the incredible life that you are meant to. You can put this book down and brush aside what you've just learnt, or you can make the stand right now to embrace the idea of who you really are. You've been working towards your purpose you're entire life. You awareness will bring newfound power to your journey.

Most importantly, remember that the means to fulfilling your purpose is a journey, not a destination. Rather than focusing on a place in your life that you want to get to, enjoy every moment, every struggle and every success that you endure along your journey. After all, life is about finding meaning, fulfillment and love, not the destination that you end at. Take baby steps every single day and you will be proud to discover miraculous advancement.

Make it your goal is to connect to Universal Energy as much as possible. When you do this you can then shine yourself brightly upon the world with the knowledge that inspiration, enthusiasm, creativity and passion will lead you to create greatness moment to moment. All of these moments will connect together to ensure that you are in love with life in the present moment and that the future you are creating **right now** will be something very special. You don't need to be anxious or fearful about the future; know deep within your heart that you're creating an amazing world for yourself and others with every moment that you chose to live in integrity with your highest values.

I've given you the roadmap; the rest is up to you. Trust me, the journey towards fulfilling your purpose is incredibly rewarding. You're a divine, unique, extraordinary person. Within you lies power beyond comprehension. Universal Energy wants certain things to happen and it has created you so that you may bring its wishes to life. Open yourself to what a far greater power is trying to create for this planet, not what you want as an individual. The world is relying on you to give it what you were created for. I wish you much happiness, love and satisfaction along your journey.

I would love to continue sharing your journey. Please don't hesitate to email me at **james@thewellbeingrevolution.com**.

About James McWhinney

To say that I've had an incredible journey over the past 10 years is a massive understatement. I've gone from being arrested, kicked out of school, money hungry, selfish, unhappy, anxious, fearful and insecure and then turned it all around to become a philosophising, life loving, meditating, spiritual, giving, caring, ultra healthy, on purpose human being. You'd be hard pressed to find a happier person living on this earth.

I've got an intense passion for helping others to live their greatest lives through striving to fulfill their greatest potentialities. My vision is to help people all over the world to live happier, more loving and more fulfilled lives.

I've written this book because I know that by fulfilling your highest potentialities you *will* enjoy increased happiness, love, fulfillment and satisfaction in your life. It is my aim to provide you with useful information that will help you to start living a life of purpose immediately. That is why this book emphasises practice rather than theory. My goal in writing this book is to help you discover your *true self*, including your greatest passions, strengths and values so that you can find more meaning, bliss and peace in your life. Within this book you will find what will truly allow you to live a life of consistent happiness and empower you to live the life that you're truly meant to live with your unique inner potential fully realized.

CPSIA information can be obtained at www.ICGtesting.com
Printed in the USA
LVOW111458120212

268311LV00002B/2/P